The Virtual Hospital

Paul Grant

The Virtual Hospital

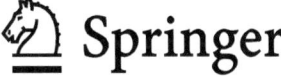 Springer

Paul Grant
Mountfield, UK

ISBN 978-3-031-69943-6   ISBN 978-3-031-69944-3   (eBook)
https://doi.org/10.1007/978-3-031-69944-3

This Springer imprint is published by the registered company Springer Nature Switzerland AG
The registered company address is: Gewerbestrasse 11, 6330 Cham, Switzerland

If disposing of this product, please recycle the paper.

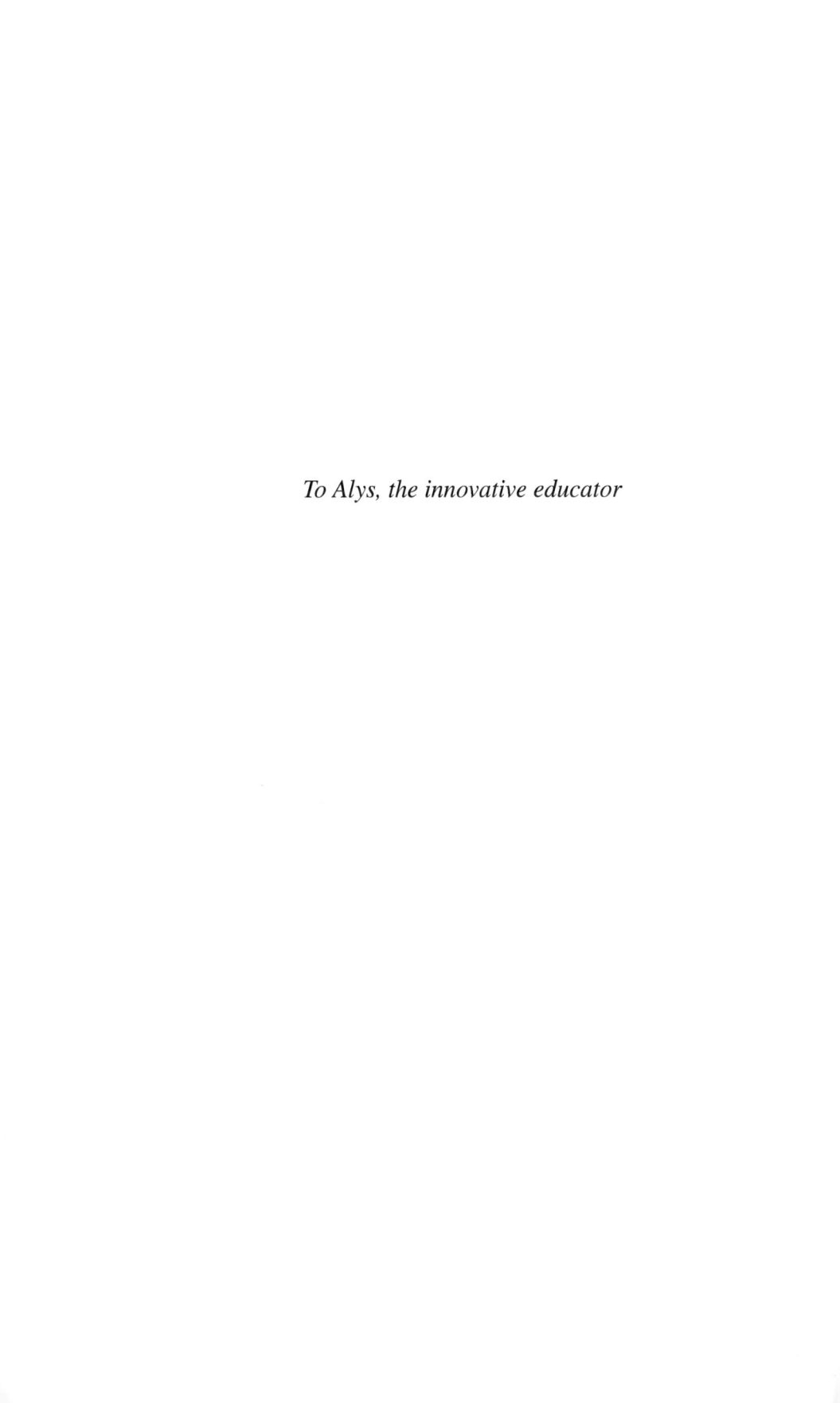

To Alys, the innovative educator

Foreword

Paul Grant has assembled this book in a way that captures the current mood of wanting to transform the traditional way of delivering healthcare but to do so ethically and humanely using evidence-informed approaches. This book addresses the plethora of new technologies ranging from artificial intelligence to biohacking and provides a reasoned perspective on the rapid expansion of virtual wards. The virtual hospital reflects the author's deep understanding and unique perspective surrounding the major developments across healthcare. There are few authors who have managed to capture all the major topics affecting digital health in one book. I am sure that as you read this book, it will generate new ideas and questions for you, just as it did for me.

London, UK   Sam Shah
September 2024

Acknowledgements

Many thanks for the support and encouragement of my colleagues who discussed the contents, hot topics, and latest developments and kept me up to date and on my toes and reviewed various elements of the manuscript.

Contents

About the Author

Dr Paul Grant is a former clinician by background, having worked in health services around the world, and latterly in the field of digital health, developing intelligent hospitals and healthcare systems for the future. He is a graduate of the University of Edinburgh's Medical Law and Ethics Master's degree course and is the author of the Gestational Diabetes Survival Guide.

Chapter 1
Introduction

"Digital technology is shaping history. But there is also the sense that it is running away with us. Where will it take us? Will our dignity and rights be enhanced or diminished? Will our societies become more equal or less equal?"

António Guterres, UN Secretary General [1]

Abstract The traditional hospital model and the way that healthcare systems work is rife with problematic legacy issues. Hospitals as institutions frequently fail to meet current challenges, societal and economic pressures, and ultimately let patients and healthcare professionals down. Arguably, many of the *wicked* problems that are endemic to health services can be tackled through 'clinical-digital transformation'. This book looks at the ways in which medicine can be done differently; finding pockets of the future and supporting evidence in the present, to explore how we can use technology to better serve society's pressing needs.

Keywords Virtual hospital · Healthcare challenges · Clinical-digital transformation · Digital health · Future healthcare

What Is a Virtual Hospital?

A virtual hospital is an umbrella term for thinking about everything that can be done outside of the traditional bricks and mortar setup of a physical hospital building. It's an exploration of all the healthcare related activities that don't require you to be in the same room as a healthcare professional at the same time. It's a concept that combines digital technologies alongside a reconsideration of the way that healthcare services are operated. It provides new, alternative pathways of care, many of which are remote and asynchronous. Unlike a traditional hospital where patients are admitted and treated on-site (Fig. 1.1), a virtual hospital works primarily through virtual platforms, such as telemedicine and uses digital communication tools. In a virtual hospital, healthcare professionals can remotely assess, diagnose, treat and monitor patients through a variety of digital means. Some key components of a virtual hospital setup may include:

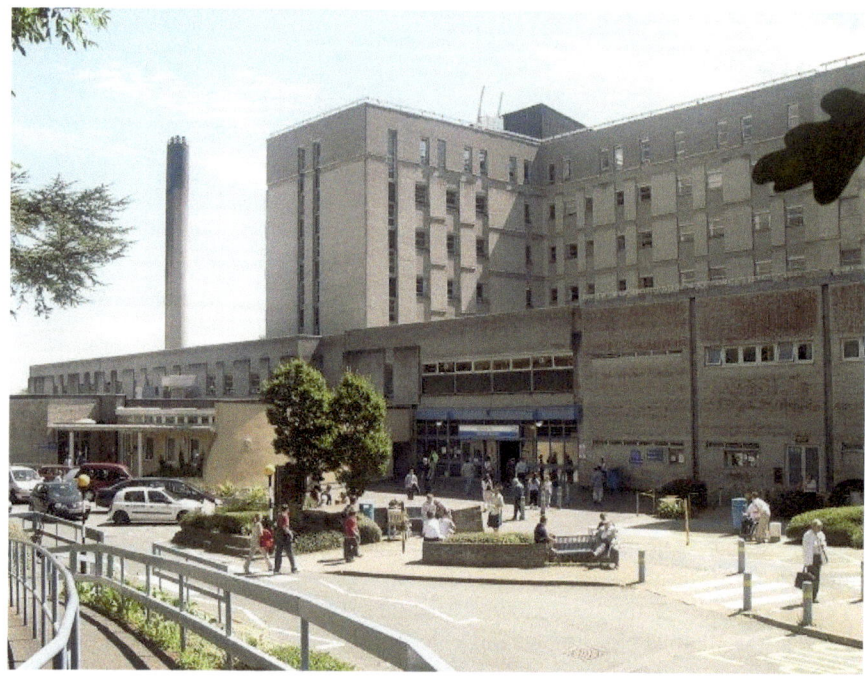

Fig. 1.1 A traditional hospital. Image Credit: Tony Atkin. Copyright: © Tony Atkin (https://www. geograph.org.uk/photo/32708). Licenced for reuse under Creative Commons license type 2.0, (unmodified). https://creativecommons.org/licenses/by-sa/2.0/

Telemedicine Two-way audio-visual communication which allows clinicians to connect with patients remotely. This type of video-conferencing means patients can consult with Doctors, discuss symptoms, receive medical advice and guidance, and communicate their concerns. The uptake of such telemedicine platforms increased significantly in light of the COVID-19 pandemic, driven by the necessity of reduced physical interaction and exposure.

Remote Monitoring The technology to record and share patient observations and vital signs has improved significantly in recent years. This may include devices that capture a patient's level of blood oxygen saturation (to indicate lung health) or a real-time sensor that captures movement (to help predict falls risk). Such digital solutions allow the transmission of health-related data from their homes to healthcare providers to allow them to monitor a patient's conditions, manage chronic illnesses, and provide timely interventions if a deterioration is identified.

Digital Health Records Electronic medical records and digital platforms are crucial in the modern healthcare era to allow the sharing, organisation and storage of patient information. Seamless access to medical records, (which contain medical histories, treatment plans, test results and medication data), for different departments and providers, as well as patients themselves, enables improved communication, cooperation and saves huge amounts of time.

Remote Diagnostics There are an increasing array of diagnostic tools and devices that enable patients to perform self-assessments or conduct medical tests at home. This might include home testing kits (blood sampling via the post), wearable glucose sensors that share their data to the cloud, or connected medical devices, such as cardiac monitors that alert the patient and clinician to abnormal heart rhythms.

Electronic Prescribing The move from a paper based, wet-signature reliant process of prescription writing, to a secure digital system has multiple benefits. Patients can receive prescription orders direct to their local pharmacy or even have medication delivered direct to their homes.

The purpose of a virtual hospital is ultimately to improve accessibility, convenience and efficiency in modern healthcare delivery, especially for patients in remote areas, individuals with mobility limitations, or those struggling with access to specialised care. By leveraging technology, virtual hospitals aim to improve patient outcomes and experience, reduce unnecessary in-person hospital visits, and optimise healthcare resources.

Drivers in the Current Healthcare Climate

In July 2024, the newly elected secretary of state for Health in the UK, Wes Streeting, declared 'The NHS is broken'. Patients are not getting the service or the care they need. There are multiple drivers to challenge and change the way that medical care is currently being delivered. Examples include the increasing demands of an ageing population replete with multiple medical problems (people are not only living longer but accumulating more problems along the way); broken health service capacity; reduced Doctor recruitment and staff retention; and following the COVID-19 pandemic there are now millions of people on hospital waiting list backlogs [2].

Whilst the use of technology and new ways of working open all sorts of possibilities for advanced healthcare delivery, we mustn't forget the caring nature of medicine and the importance of human interactions. It's this tension that needs to be constantly borne in mind before getting too carried away with smart and sexy technology. Furthermore, we are now living in an age where the role of Doctors has shifted socio-culturally from the friendly and avuncular family Doctor who looks after you and your relatives from cradle to grave, to that of technicians, specialist and 'ologists', who fix disparate issues in a transactional manner (much like taking your car in for a fanbelt replacement) without the traditional holistic aspects of care. There is frequently an idealised view of how we *should* be cared for when we become unwell, that society can no longer realistically deliver. With this is mind it makes sense to look at the issues with the present situation so that we can consider how to deliver medical care differently.

In this book, I would like to take you on a tour of the many interesting and varied ways that medicine can be, could be, and will be, delivered in the new ways in the years to come, from virtual wards and clinics, to artificial intelligence, biohacking and beyond.

We first need to consider the current structure and issues around current health-care delivery in the developed world and recognise that the general set-up around how people access healthcare and the ways in which their care is managed tend to fall into similar patterns in many westernised nations. We'll look at what we actually mean by 'healthcare', what counts as a hospital, what do Doctors do, and ask if we are using them as effectively as we could be (spoiler alert—no we're not). I then want to demonstrate how the foundations have been laid for shifting clinical work out of hospitals into the online sphere, through the utilisation of both virtual in-patient and virtual out-patient services, a course of action spurred on significantly by the global pandemic in 2020 [3]. Following this, what are the options for other applications of remote medical care? Recent years have already seen a con-certed shift to online primary care to circumvent the dearth of primary care access, but what about emergency medicine and other fields—is this possible?

As we become more sophisticated in our tech monitoring and disease screening, we also need to look at the realm of proactive care—picking up on diseases before the patient is even aware they are ill, as well as the use of trackers, wearables and apps to nudge people into better habits, behaviours and lifestyles [4]. Emerging technological advances suggest that the virtual personal trainer/nutritionist and life-style guru is not far away.

Finally, we need to discuss whether this is the right direction of travel. It may seem cool, futuristic and smart to contemplate the ways in which healthcare could be revolutionised through the use of technology (it may certainly help to signifi-cantly improve outcomes and reduce variation in care and accessibility), but along-side this we have to consider the safety, the ethics, the equitability and the philosophical principles around virtual medicine [5]. What might we lose in terms of personal care and autonomy whilst Silicon Valley tech giants make a fast buck? The majority of people who go into the caring professions, don't tend to do it for the money, it's a vocation, but there are currently many systemic barriers which impede healthcare professionals to do their jobs well. Hopefully many of these new techno-logical solutions will help to augment clinician's work and improve their working lives, enhancing their interactions with patients, rather than turn medicine into a faceless, transactional production line (Fig. 1.2). Technology advances in healthcare are frequently great but only when caring humanity remains at the forefront of all considerations.

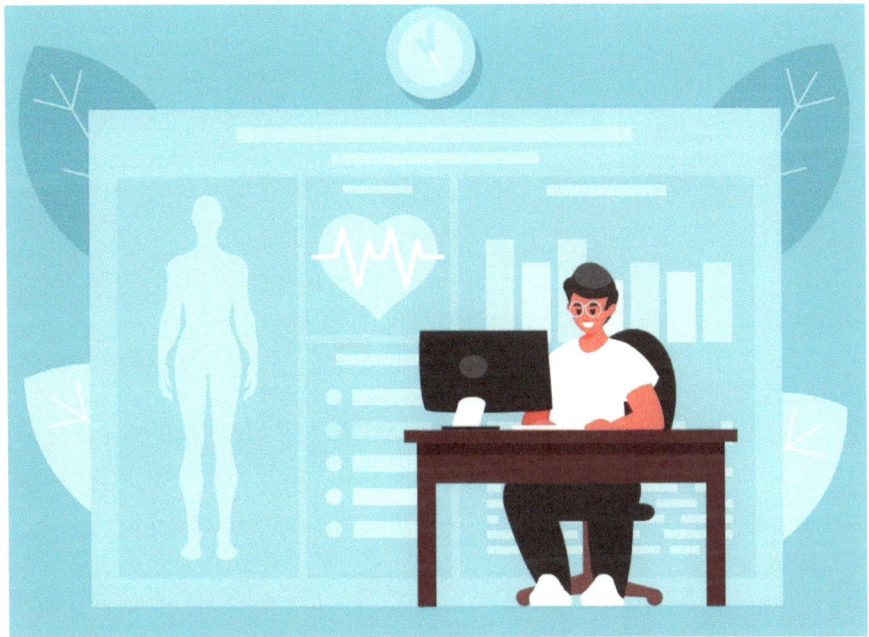

Fig. 1.2 The virtual medicine future. Source: Free vectors.net, unmodified (https://free-vectors. net/healthcare/computer-diagnostics-of-health). Licenced for reuse under Creative Commons license type 4.0. https://creativecommons.org/licenses/by/4.0/

References

1. Guterres A. UN Secretary General's roadmap for digital cooperation. 2019. https://www. un.org/en/content/digital-cooperation-roadmap/#:~:text=UNITED%20NATIONS%20SECR ETARY%2DGENERAL&text=%E2%80%9CDigital%20technology%20is%20shaping%20 history,rights%20be%20enhanced%20or%20diminished%3F. Accessed 10 Jun 2024.
2. Morris J, Reed S. How much is Covid-19 to blame for growing NHS waiting times? QualityWatch: Nuffield Trust and Health Foundation. 2022. https://www.nuffieldtrust.org. uk/resource/how-much-is-covid-19-to-blame-for-growing-nhs-waiting-times. Accessed 15 Jul 2023.
3. World Health Organisation. COVID-19 has caused major disruptions and backlogs in health care, new WHO study finds. 2022. https://www.who.int/europe/news/item/20-07-2022-covid-19-has-caused-major-disruptions-and-backlogs-in-health-care%2D%2Dnew-who-study-finds. Accessed 15 Jul 2023.
4. Shaver J. The state of telehealth before and after the COVID-19 pandemic. Prim Care. 2022;49(4):517–30.
5. World Health Organization, OECD, International Bank for Reconstruction and Development/ The World Bank. Delivering quality health services: a global imperative for universal health coverage. Geneva; 2018. ISBN 978-92-4-151390-6.

Chapter 2
Challenging the Paradigm of Healthcare Delivery

Abstract It's vital to understand the current model of health and care provision and balance this with the knowledge that it is struggling to cope with unprecedented demands. This leads to inadequate service provision and detriments to patient care. There are multiple barriers and pain points that exist within health systems that limit their ability to provide the care that people need and that clinicians want to deliver. This chapter explores what is 'healthcare', what is a hospital and what is it that Doctors actually do, before making the case for change.

Keywords Healthcare challenges · Health service burden · Waiting lists · Elective care · Hospitals · Primary care

The Status Quo

The current model of healthcare is largely based around face-to-face interactions in a setting deemed appropriate to an individual patient's need (or more commonly, the clinician's convenience). If you are suffering from an acute problem such as a sore throat, then you might go to see your family Doctor (or primary care physician) in a general practice setting (often described as primary care) (Fig. 2.1). If you were experiencing serious digestive problems, then you would see a specialist Gastroenterologist in the local hospital (secondary care) who may investigate and manage your problems over a prolonged period. And if you were unfortunate enough to have a rarer or significant and difficult to manage condition, for example needing a heart and lung transplant, then you would be looked after in a 'tertiary' care setting such as the National Hospital for Neurology and Neurosurgery at Queen's Square in London or the Memorial Sloan Kettering Cancer Centre in New York. This system sorts people into the category that is most suited to them and where the most appropriate resources sit.

Unfortunately, there are problems in terms of capacity and organisation at each of these levels. Anyone who has tried to get an appointment with their primary care Doctor in recent years will recognise that it is a battle to even get past the

P. Grant, *The Virtual Hospital*, https://doi.org/10.1007/978-3-031-69944-3_2

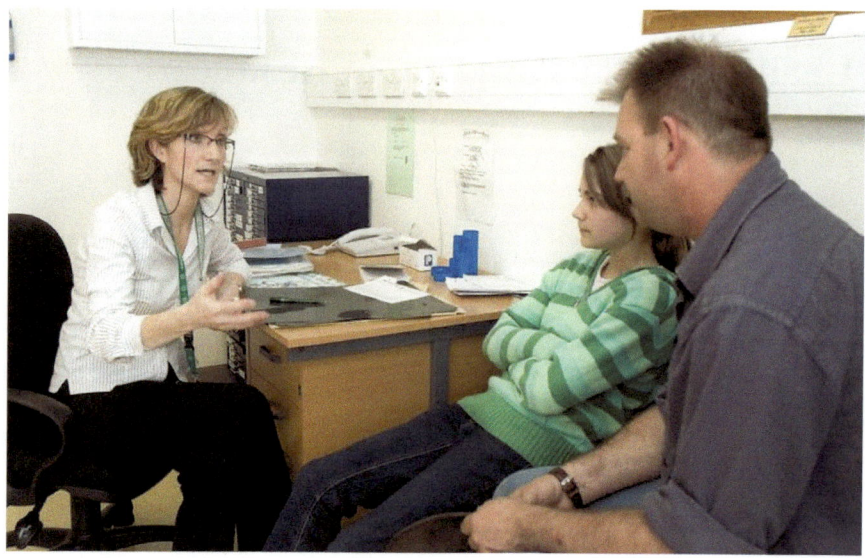

Fig. 2.1 A traditional Doctor–Patient consultation. Image Credit—CMRF Crumlin (Source: https://www.flickr.com/photos/cmrf_crumlin/4838022938/in/photostream/).   Unmodified. Licenced for reuse under Creative Commons license type 2.0. https://creativecommons.org/licenses/by/2.0/

receptionists (the true gatekeepers of healthcare) and schedule an appointment. When you do, it is commonly '*one appointment, one problem*' as it is hard for the beleaguered clinician to deal with much beyond this in the standard 10-min slot. You may get passed to a lower grade of clinician such as a nurse practitioner or a paramedic for them to deal with you instead and they can hopefully diagnose and manage you via a protocolised pathway, only escalating to the Doctor when there are problems.

The rates of burnout and early retirement amongst family Doctors are significant and repeated Government promises of thousands of new clinicians are slow to be realised. In the US, primary care physicians work in a fragmented, underfunded system, "hobbled by widespread inequities and chronic workforce shortages, with an uneven distribution of providers and a medical education system that holds primary care in low esteem" [1].

Speak to any primary care Doctor and it is hard to find a happy and content practitioner that is master of their domain. At the time of writing there is a commission underway to review the entire nature of general practice in the United Kingdom, with threats to nationalise primary care. It will be fascinating to see if they are able to assess it both realistically and apolitically. Aneurin Bevan, when reforming healthcare in the 1940s, famously had to 'stuff their mouths with gold' to bring General Practitioners on board and work alongside new the national health service.

When patients are referred to see a specialist from primary care, the process for getting seen, can be tortuous and prolonged. Waiting lists for specialist out-patient services (which can involve anything from Cardiology to ENT services) are at an all-time high, over 7 million in total, with over a third of a million people waiting longer than a year for treatment in the UK [2].

After a wait of many months, you may finally get to see a Consultant or Registrar (Doctor in training), during this time your medical problems may have progressed significantly (or alternatively cleared up by themself), and the clinician has to essentially work you up from scratch, organise investigations, gather further information, review your records, and decide on a management plan for you. If you need to start a course of medication, the Consultant has to write (yes write by letter) to your primary care Doctor to ask them if they wouldn't mind awfully writing a prescription for you, which adds to treatment delays. If you need an intervention, for example a radiological procedure such as an angioplasty or even surgery, then you have another big wait on your hands. Secondary care struggles because it also has capacity and demand management problems. Fill rates for new Consultant posts were at only 48% in 2021. The number of GP referrals to Consultant-led outpatient services that were unsuccessful because there were no slots available has jumped by 87% between February 2020 and November 2021—a staggering increase.

This prolongation of waiting times leads to further problems, not only deterioration in the health status of the patiently waiting patient, but also pressure on the primary care Doctor to manage cases outside of their comfort zone and expertise, putting patients at risk and struggling to manage expectations, scheduling more follow up visits to keep an eye on them and contributing to burnout, frustration, and stress due to the additional burdens placed on them. Illustrative quotes from an interesting Canadian study by Marshall et al. on the problems of specialist waiting times include "*I've found that you have to beg to be considered to be seen*", and "*I do not refer anyone to GI as it gives patients false hope that they ever would be seen*", which makes for uncomfortable reading [3].

These problems are exacerbated by the rather old-fashioned outpatient model that is arguable very inefficient (for both patients and Doctors) and cannot flex easily to meet surges in demand or function in new ways (Fig. 2.2). Something as simple as organising diagnostic tests prior to a patient physically attending an outpatient clinic are still an anathema to many hospital clinics. The Doctors themselves are not to blame for this. It reflects a system that was built to cope with a different set of problems in a different time and sadly hospital bureaucracy and managerialism can make it hard for hospitals to adapt.

The traditional solutions to the problem of rising healthcare needs include disease prevention, public health measures, education, hiring more staff (often from abroad), and trying to manage expectations. These fixes are often not implemented effectively or don't work sufficiently well anymore. New ways are desperately needed to disrupt current systems and change the paradigm of healthcare as much as we can, in order to address current and future needs. This could involve anything from encouraging greater patient self-management (the monitored self), facilitating greater doctor productivity, harnessing digital technologies to streamline care, to building a networked hospital in the cloud. Ultimately this book is about challenging long standing assumptions about 'how we do healthcare' and not being afraid to

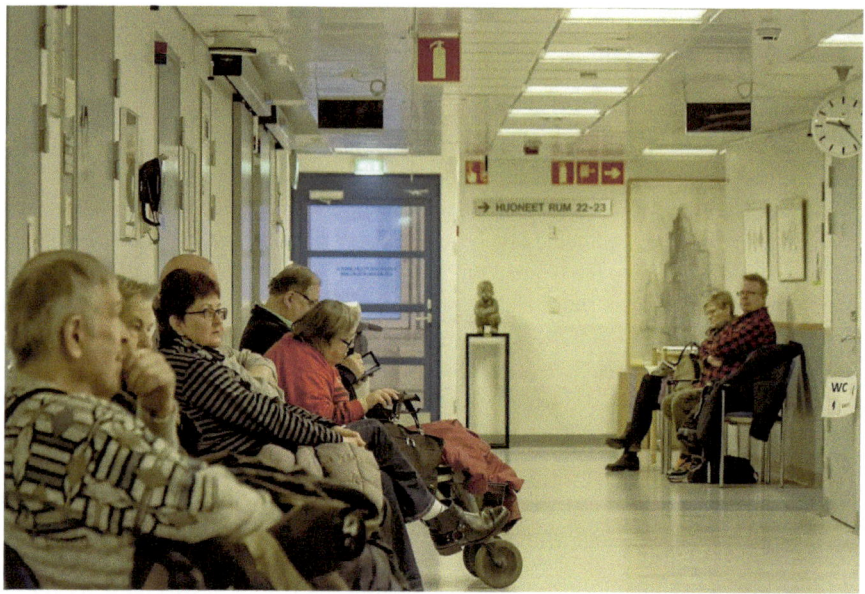

Fig. 2.2 A traditional clinic waiting area. Image Credit: Jori Samonen. (Unmodified from source: https://pxhere.com/en/photo/294710). Licenced for reuse under Creative Commons license type 2.0. https://creativecommons.org/licenses/by/2.0/

take down some sacred cows. Everyone will agree that the healthcare institutions and healthcare professionals work extremely hard, but they face resource poor conditions and have to fight for their patients. Shockingly, '*corridor medicine*' is now arising as a new speciality in its own right. The UK NHS is a fantastic institution, greatly admired across the world, but it is a clunky and uncoordinated beast, a political football and not set up for the demands of the twenty-first century. Can we explore how we might do things better?

What Is Healthcare?

Healthcare is the organised provision of medical care to individuals or communities by medical professionals, in order to restore our physical or mental wellbeing—'the maintenance or improvement of health via the prevention, diagnosis and treatment of disease, illness and injury'. There are multiple objectives under this banner, which broadly speaking should be;

1. **To reduce the burden of disease across the whole population** i.e. minimising illness and death, to alleviate suffering and to (hopefully) increase people's quality of life. This has to be done in a proportional way, focussing the greatest amount of resource on the problems that cause the most harm—which means an

understanding of rationing and cost-effectiveness. We are very fortunate to have institutions such as NICE in the UK (the National Institute for Health and Clinical Excellence) and programmes such GIRFT (Getting It Right First Time) which had its origins in the US, that help us to understand and implement the evidence base for our efforts.

2. **To deliver said healthcare safely and in a high-quality fashion** i.e. minimising the risk of clinical errors [4], reducing variation in care (not everyone gets treated the same because of disparities in the system and individual clinician and organisational differences) and increasing adherence to best practice (it's important to recognise that medicine is still shifting from an artform to a standardised recipe—there is much to consider when it comes to balancing frenesis (practical wisdom) with the evidence base).

3. **To be patient centered, inclusive and responsive.** Currently healthcare is heavily oriented around systems and processes and less so on the patient experience. What is convenient and useful for clinicians and hospitals is not always the same for those we serve.

With these overarching aims in mind, there are a spectrum of considerations that follow. At one end a belief that we should be able to provide detailed, holistic, personalised healthcare for everyone over their whole life course—to the other extreme—that an illness or a presenting complaint or a disease entity, is a discrete problem that just needs to be fixed or ameliorated, and then the individual patient discharged on their own recognisance. Whilst I am an advocate of the former and the latter seems less caring and comprehensive, we realistically need to understand that a compromise needs to be found somewhere between the two.

Fully individualised and holistic healthcare is arguably an aspirational luxury that we have been struggling to provide for years and can ill-afford to sustain at a societal level. People have fond memories of the so-called Dr. Finlay fallacy[1] and this really can't be achieved unless you want to seek private medical care.[2] So how best to address the challenges of care delivery on a large scale to meet our three objectives?

---

[1] AJ. Cronin's fictional hero Dr. John Finlay (a series of books and then a television series) was set in the 1930's and relayed the exploits of a young idealist Scottish GP attempting to modernise medical practice. He is a charming character and gets to know his patients very well over the years, it is his trademark to provide a continuous relationship. A key tenet of the Doctor–Patient relationship is the bond of trust, communication and respect that we all desire and is best for patient care. The unfortunate fallacy is that this relationship does not exist anymore. Everyone is supposed to have a named primary care Doctor, but it is hard to ever get to see them. Doctors don't have the time or the headspace to get to know their patients and their families properly. Serial locums prop up general practice and rates of GP burnout are at an all-time high.

[2] Just to be clear one does not wish to advocate privatisation in the received sense, or the disastrous US model of healthcare which is both ineffective and immoral at the same time. However, there is now a marked rise in the types and numbers of private medical practitioners, everything from lifestyle GP's to health concierges, seeking to profit from the frustrations of accessing publicly provided healthcare.

Top-down re-organisation of health services is often ineffective because it does not tackle the underlying contributing factors. The dream of increasing capacity (more Doctors and Nurses) does not work, as it takes many years to recruit and train new clinicians. Stealing the best talent from elsewhere in the world does continue but remains ethically questionable. We can do little to reduce the demands on the health service—people are living longer with more problems and expectations are much higher as patients become more consumerist in their approach. You can out-source services to the independent sector to a certain degree, but it is expensive and unpopular in a country that counts the NHS as *it's national religion*, plus the fact that private Hospitals themselves are struggling with capacity and more and more patients are now self-funding their own operations abroad, travelling to the EU for surgery through organisations such as My Medical Gateway International.

There is option of promoting greater patient self-care and responsibility through supported programmes such as DESMOND (Diabetes Education and Self-Management for Ongoing and Newly diagnosed type 2 Diabetes) or the C-PEP (COPD Patient Education Programme), which enables patients to take more ownership of their long-term medical conditions, but this still needs to be done via a Consultant led multi-disciplinary team and is not an adequate replacement for everything that is required for chronic disease care. Preventative medicine, education and screening programmes all have a role to play, but we are still left with a heavy volume of unwell people needing medical attention and insufficient numbers of Dr. Finlay's to go around. The issue is that we cannot sustainably deliver effective healthcare as things stand at this pivotal moment in our history.

A Hospital. What Is It?

The oldest Hospitals in the UK, Bart's and St. Thomas', both in London, date back to the 12th century and have their origins in the simple need to bring sick patients together into a setting where they could be cared for by nursing and medical staff (even if it was only for bloodletting and enemas). Their condition can be monitored, treatments administered, and their response assessed. This physical consolidation makes practical sense. Over time, this Hospital model has evolved to incorporate out-patient clinics (run by the Hospital Doctor who would mainly be looking after in-patients, but whom has a special interest in a particular area of medicine, for instance Gynaecology) to help treat people not ill enough to require in-patient admission, therapy departments (such as rehabilitation), radiology and pathology departments, operating theatres, emergency departments (a relatively new phenomenon), dialysis units, diabetes centres, linear accelerators, helicopter pads and so on, in order to maximise propinquity. By having all your healthcare resources in one place you are able to provide connected care and services efficiently at scale—economies of concentration.

The downsides of this centralisation though are multiple; if you don't live near a hospital, access is difficult, especially if a merged hospital trust decides to shut down the maternity units on one of its sites and patients have to travel long distances to get care. This means disproportionately reduced access to care in remote and rural communities (so called distance decay). Even if you live close to a hospital, getting there, parking and taking time off work are major inconveniences and out-patient services are notoriously Doctor rather than patient centric (need to be reviewed for your thyroid condition 4 weeks after starting treatment? *Sorry, no come back in 4 months on a Wednesday morning. If you miss your appointment, you'll be discharged*).

Additional problems that hospitals face are that they are hives for the spread of diseases such as clostridium difficile and norovirus (who would have thought that ramming a building full of sick and frail people would cause problems), they are dangerous (the clinical risk associated with being in a hospital is high, this could be anything from a medication error to having the wrong type of surgery). Secondary care related adverse drug reactions for example leads to longer hospital stays cost-ing the NHS £14.8 million and causing or contributing to 1081 deaths annually, according to the Manchester Centre for Health Economics. In the US, rates of medi-cal errors in Hospitals are significant. Researchers led by Dr. Martin Makary of the Johns Hopkins University School of Medicine, found that based on a total of 35,416,020 hospitalisations, there was a pooled incidence rate of 251,454 deaths per year—or about 9.5% of all deaths—that stemmed from medical error [5].

Fragmented care on busy wards is dangerous and the system does not work effectively because at the end of a patient's journey, after they have been fixed up and stabilised, they remain trapped and vulnerable in Hospital by inadequate social services provision (the so-called bed blockers), leading to the recurrent news stories that we see where ambulances have to queue outside of the Emergency Department for hours on end, because Hospital throughput has ground to a halt. Hospital ser-vices have markedly long waiting times exacerbated by chronic underfunding. The one size fits all model does not seem to work well across the board, with increasing numbers of healthcare commissioners having to set up satellite clinics and commu-nity services or out-source operations to the private sector to increase capacity. The Jurassic culture of Hospital trusts are slow to adapt, and innovation is not promoted, because of the dislike of change. New ideas are often shot down with more speed and vigour than an Orthopod's hammer. Meanwhile Doctors complain about prac-tising *'battlefield medicine'* in *'third world conditions'* whilst trying to provide care.

Historically, we have passively accepted particular characteristics of Hospitals structure and organisation which have conditioned us to believe that a Hospital must behave and operate in a certain way. Acute hospitals frequently have priority in spending plans but arguably this may not be the best investment for health gain. We need to search for more good evidence on the costs and feasibility of alternative models of care than is currently available because we don't have the capacity, resources, and skills to continue as things currently are.

What Is a Doctor?

To train a medical professional up to the level of full qualification takes up to 6 years and has societal costs of around $1.1 million dollars to put them through medical school in the US and roughly £250,000 of taxpayers money in the UK. However, these junior Doctors then require numerous additional years of training (4 in the context of Primary Care physicians and anywhere from 6 to 10 years for medical and surgical specialists) to be properly independent and autonomous practitioners (Fig. 2.3). In some places this is flexible. Whilst working in New Zealand I was amused by adverts in the Doctors mess for the local accelerated training scheme for GP's which had a total duration of 32 weeks before full qualification, such was the heightened demand.

Our present system of medical care, based on a rigid division between the Hospital service and primary care, is the product of many historical events; the rapid development of outpatient departments in the nineteenth century was probably one of the most important. Traditionally, the existence of two separate classes of Doctor, provided a good opportunity for charging patients more money. Initial assessment by a family Doctor to receive a potential diagnosis, followed by the need to see a specialist for dedicated management is a form of supplier-induced demand. We now have perpetuated this system and have around 40 specialities and sub-specialities of medicine and surgery, undertaking increasingly complex patient care. A major issue facing the medical profession (and by extension the general public) is that the fill rates for Consultant posts in many specialities are at an all-time low. The graph below (Fig. 2.4), based on OECD data shows the average number of Doctors per 1000 population, with the average across OECD countries being 3.7, and 3.1 in the UK respectively.

This has been exacerbated by a multitude of problems including poor workforce planning, high burnout (rates of depression, alcoholism, divorce and suicide remain higher than the population average), pension and tax problems, the gnawing effects of bureaucracy and the sheer exhausting grind of having to work harder than ever

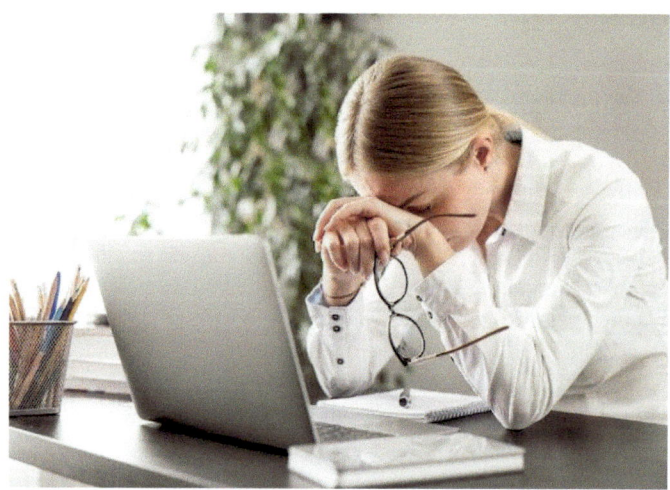

Fig. 2.3 Doctor burnout. Image credit: Designed by Freepik (Source: https://www.freepik.com/ free-photo/side-view-woman-having-headache-before-class_9021856.htm#query=tired%20 doctor&position=6&from_view=search&track=ais&uuid=a51f6 4ec-1bb9-49ea-a3e0-58fe81703922)

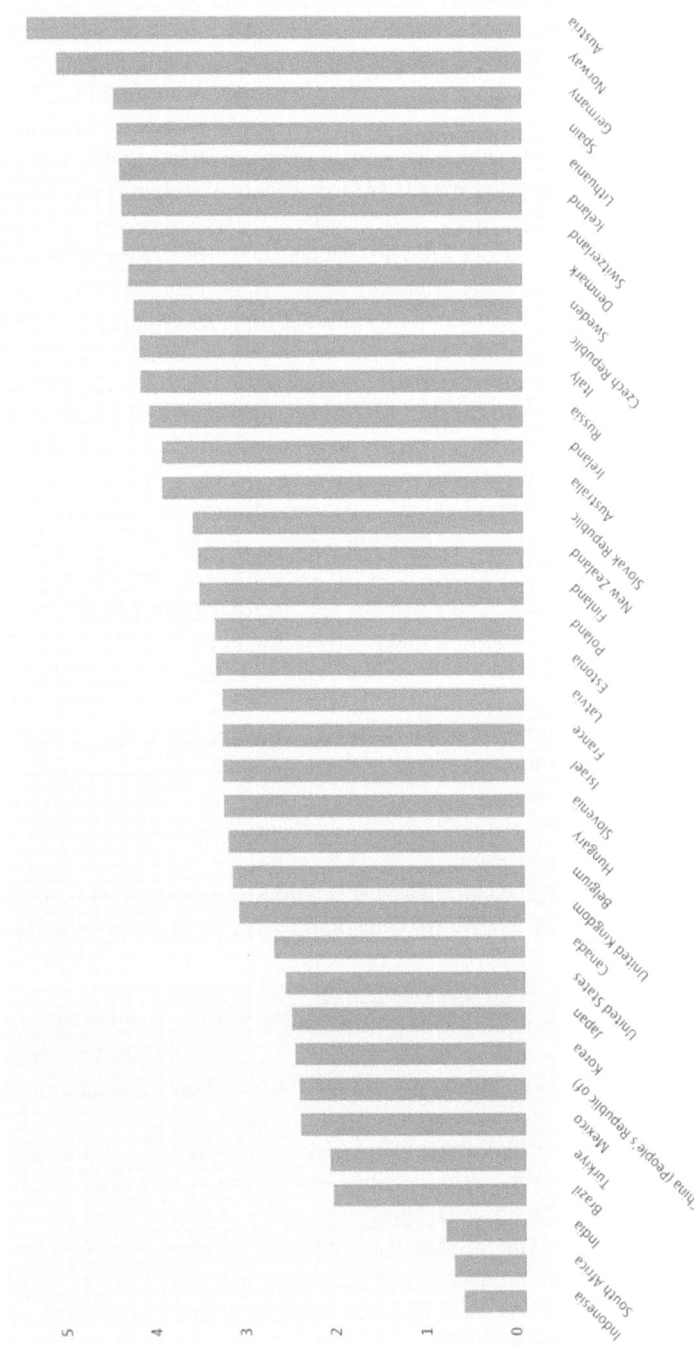

Fig. 2.4 Graph of OECD countries showing the average numbers of Doctors per 1000 head of population. Image Source: OECD (2024), "Doctors" (indicator), https://doi.org/10.1787/4355e1ec-en. Open Access—All data, reports and analysis in all formats are now available under an open licence, allowing users to freely access, use, translate, and share the Organisation's work

before. The European Working Time Directive did help reduce the pressure on the long hours worked by junior Doctors in the EU, but this simply meant that the work was shifted onto those who were exempt—the senior Doctors, who in their middle age were less equipped to deal with frequent, long on-calls and now have less support, given the breakdown of the traditional firm structure. Additionally, Consultant specialists are inequitably distributed around countries. There are regions that have perpetually unfilled posts because they are in unattractive locations, and nobody wants to spend their career (after over ten or more years of training) in a low status locale (apologies to Grimsby) [6].

In terms of what a Doctor does day to day, and what they were trained for at medical school and in their early years, there is a significant disparity. You may think that a Consultant spends the majority of their time undertaking ward rounds, talking to relatives and seeing people in out-patient clinics, but the reality of what constitutes an 'essential Doctor function' is relatively limited. By this I mean the absolute core essence of what Doctors do (assess, investigate, diagnose and treat people). Clinicians have an amazing ability to process and synthesize information and based on knowledge (long lists of potential causes of each and every presenting complaint), experience, pattern recognition (thousands of hours of doing the same thing over and over), judgement and decision making, (think of the many examinations a Doctor has to pass throughout their career, not just to pass, but to excel at) they will know exactly, in almost any given situation, what to do. These are the brilliant things that Doctors do and are rightly lauded for. However, this is not what a twenty-first century Doctor spends the bulk of their time doing. They in fact spend a rather large amount of time emailing each other or their managers, logging onto multiple clunky IT systems, chasing results, attending meetings, undertaking administrative tasks, business planning, performing audits, managing their peers and complaining about how little they are being listened to, living in a bureaucracy that they do not understand and feel powerless to change, when all they want to do is deliver better care for their patients.

For those clinicians in procedure-based specialities i.e. the interventional cardiologists and surgeons, the relative amount of time spent physically cutting into people is surprisingly low, this is because operating theatre processes are inefficient and result in Doctors sitting around doing very little for long periods of time, or managing their sidegigs on their iPhones whilst they wait for patients to be wheeled in and out. There are even now niche companies (such as Xyla Elective recovery) who recognise that optimising theatre time usage is a whole business opportunity in itself [7].

All of this would seem like a massively distracting anathema to those twelfth century Doctors at Barts who were probably very efficient with their leeches (as they did not have much else to work with). At a strike, if you stopped all Doctors having to respond to their emails, then the health of the nation would go up massively because of increased productivity. It's not that such extraneous tasks are not important, but we shouldn't be using our most precious resource to do such a large amount of administration or hinder their ability to work by taking away their secretaries. Ultimately, we are not taking optimal advantage of our highly skilled and

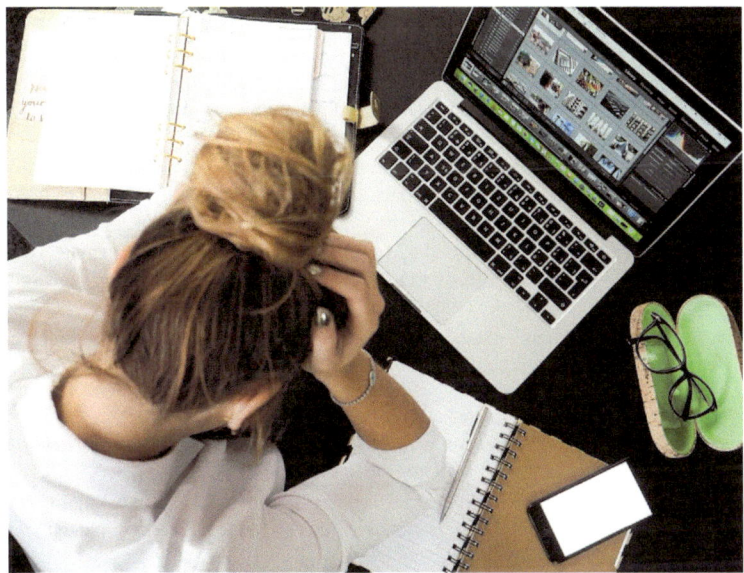

Fig. 2.5 Stressed Doctor. Image Source: Rawpixel. (unmodified from https://www.rawpixel.com/ image/5926536). Licenced for reuse under Creative Commons license type 0. https://creativecommons.org/publicdomain/zero/1.0/

well-paid medical workforce (Fig. 2.5). There are so many distractions, blockers and low-level annoyances that get in the way of them doing their core Doctoring functions that it renders many of our care pathways ineffective and slow as a consequence.

The Case for Change

The problems and challenges facing the provision of good medical care broadly relate to the massively increased demand on health services, the ageing population, the rise in multi-morbidity, the expensive nature of healthcare delivery, disparity and inequality in the provision of care, accessibility, rising stress and burnout in the medical and nursing workforce, high levels of medical errors and failure to successfully leverage the benefits of technology or to transform outdated working practices.

The change equation is a well-recognised tool that highlights how the process of change can be initiated (Table 2.1) [8]. It comprises; $C = A \times B \times D > R$

C = the change that you wish to bring about
A = dissatisfaction with the status quo
B = the vision for the desired future state
D = the first practical steps required to brings about a change
R = resistance or barriers to the change that must be overcome

Table 2.1 Elements of the 'change equation' in the context of early twenty-first century healthcare systems

Desired change (C)	Improved care delivery and quality, reduced costs, increased efficiency and convenience, enhanced patient and healthcare worker satisfaction and experience.
Dissatisfaction with the status quo (A)	Massive waiting lists, vast healthcare spend, problems with recruitment and retention of clinicians, detriments to quality of care, negative experiences.
Vision for the future state (B)	A well organised and supportive system of healthcare delivery that takes advantage of digital solutions to transform care pathways in an organised, equitable and patient centred approach.
First steps to bring about change (D)	An understanding of care pathways and how new technologies can overcome pain points and blockers. Stakeholder engagement to review areas for change and acceptability of new processes and pathways. Local, regional, national change management and organisational development approaches.
Resistance to change (R)	Negative perceptions or misunderstanding of what technologies can do. General resistance/entrenchment against any form of change (fear of the unknown, risk aversion). Cultural and behavioural factors. Lack of leadership and support. Limited resources. Complex regulatory environment.

We're clear on A (dissatisfaction with the status quo), people definitely want C (change for the better), what we need to work on is the future vision (B), and how to make a start (D) in order to climb over the mountain of R!

Whilst change is clearly needed, successful change implementation in the health service requires recognising and addressing the barriers through careful planning, stakeholder engagement, leadership support, effective communication and change management, as well as commitment to continuous improvement.

Next Steps

To summarise where we are now, it appears as though we are trying to do too much with too little. Our healthcare system is disjointed and both Hospitals and the medical profession run along antiquated and unproductive lines. In the rest of this book, I am going to explore potentially different ways of doing things whilst bearing in mind that not only are people uncomfortable with change of any sort, but when you start introducing terms such as 'clinical algorithms' or 'virtual consultations', there can be a reflex response of immediate judgement and reluctance to engage. This is not the case here, I'm unafraid to challenge the fact that things should be done better, if that means looking at things from a new and interesting perspective then please come and join me in the virtual Hospital.

References

1. Levins H. How can we fix primary care? Five experts discuss primary care reform in a Penn LDI Virtual Seminar. 2022. https://ldi.upenn.edu/our-work/research-updates/how-can-we-fix-primary-care/#:~:text=The%20general%20consensus%20was%20that,determinants%20 of%20health%2C%20and%20a. Accessed 27 Oct 2023.
2. NHS England. Consultant-led referral to treatment waiting times data 2022–23. https://www. england.nhs.uk/statistics/statistical-work-areas/rtt-waiting-times/rtt-data-2022-23/
3. Marshall EG, Miller L, Moritz LR. Challenges and impacts from wait times for specialist care identified by primary care providers: results from the MAAP study cross-sectional survey. Healthc Manage Forum. 2023;36(5):340–6. https://doi.org/10.1177/08404704231182671.
4. Elliott RA, Camacho E, Jankovic D, Sculpher MJ, Faria R. Economic analysis of the prevalence and clinical and economic burden of medication error in England. BMJ Qual Saf. 2021;30(2):96–105. https://doi.org/10.1136/bmjqs-2019-010206.
5. Makary MA, Daniel M. Medical error—the third leading cause of death in the US. BMJ. 2016;353:i2139. https://doi.org/10.1136/bmj.i2139.
6. Wise J. Record number of consultant physician jobs are unfilled, census shows. BMJ. 2022;378:o1782. https://doi.org/10.1136/bmj.o1782.
7. Xyla Elective recovery. https://xylaservices.com/about-xyla/. Accessed 10 Mar 2024.
8. Beckhard R, Harris RT. Organizational transitions: managing complex change, Addison-Wesley series on organization development. 1st ed. Reading, MA: Addison-Wesley Publishing; 1977.

Chapter 3
The Virtual Ward

Abstract Virtual wards are a transformative concept reshaping the landscape of healthcare delivery in the twenty-first century. They are care models designed to extend healthcare beyond the confines of traditional hospitals and clinics, facilitating patient-centric care in a digital age, on a background of growing demands on health services and the changing dynamics of healthcare delivery. This chapter explores the origins, evolution, and the impact of virtual wards on the healthcare ecosystem.

Keywords Virtual wards · Virtual hospitals · Remote monitoring · Internet of things · Referral and triage · Patient empowerment · Accessibility · Clinical-digital transformation

What Is a Virtual Ward?

When people think of a Hospital, the image is classically of a large white blocky building with an emergency department stuck on the front end and the rest being those long Nightingale wards lined with beds on either side, full of patients in pyjamas or gowns (Fig. 3.1). Trolleys being pushed back and forth. Nurses in smart, crisp uniforms. Doctors in white overcoats wearing their stethoscopes, perhaps followed by a gaggle of medical students.

The other things that you'll get in the Hospital are likely to be the X-ray department, the laboratory for the pathology tests, operating theatres and well, that's about it? What else do you need in a Hospital? Everything is consolidated for practicality and economies of scale. The out-patient department is tacked on the side as a way of dealing with reviewing patients after they've been in hospital or as a way of getting the specialist to see them without them having to be sick enough to actually be in a Hospital bed.

Let's talk about those people in the beds. The ones that the whole infrastructure is built around. The traditional patient journey—the way to get into a hospital bed is

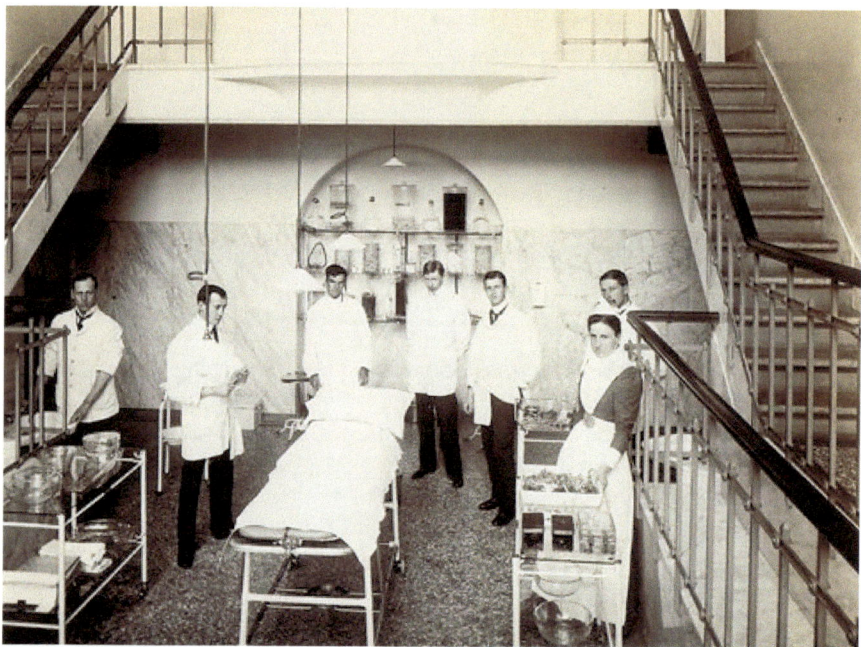

Fig. 3.1 The traditional hospital. Image Source: Look and Learn History Picture Archive (unmodified from https://www.lookandlearn.com/history-images/YW029847V/University-College-Hospital-medical-staff-in-an-operating-theatre-which-has-stairs-leading-up-on-either-side). Licenced for reuse under Creative Commons license type 4.0

through a few different routes and worth contemplating—because after all, this is a book about doing things differently.

- **The Emergency Admission**: something acute has happened to Mrs. Jones, perhaps it's a flare up of her gallstones, she calls her GP, she can't get through, feels really unwell, spikes a high temperature and gets some severe cramping abdominal pains. Because it's the worse pain she's ever felt (she's not normally one to complain) and her husband is worried, they decide to call an ambulance. The paramedics are concerned and it's clear that she needs to go to the Emergency department. She's rushed to Hospital and after a few short hours waiting outside in the ambulance bay, is finally allowed inside the building to be assessed by the on-call surgical Doctor. He pokes her abdomen, sends her for a CT scan and it's clear that she has something nasty going on. She's admitted onto the surgical ward and the plan is to give her some antibiotics, some painkillers and see how she responds. The surgical Consultant comes in to see her the following morning, pokes her again in the abdomen, looks at her discerningly over his glasses and thinks that *watchful waiting* is the best approach.

- There are two likely outcomes in this common scenario. Either things steadily improve, she responds to the 'conservative' management, or her underlying problem gets worse, and something needs to be done i.e. being taken to theatres and a bucket of pus cleared out from her abdominal cavity. Eventually after a period of recuperation/recovery/rehabilitation, Mrs. Jones gets to go home. Given the practical delays between the surgical Consultant giving the greenlight for the patient to leave and everything being organised, plus the pressures on Hospital beds, many patients may spend a day hanging about in a 'discharge lounge' being kept an eye on, whilst waiting for their TTO medications ('to take out') and their transport home.

- **The Elective Admission:** this is the far more organised and orderly way of getting into Hospital. You're already known to have a problem—likely through outpatient services, and you've got to come into Hospital to now have something done.

- Mr. Cohen's been experiencing worsening angina over the last 2 years, and he's recently had a coronary angiogram that suggests he's got rather severe narrowing of two of his coronary arteries. He has a strong family history of heart disease at a young age. If something isn't done, then he is highly likely to have a heart attack—which would be a very bad thing. He needs coronary bypass surgery but is not acutely unwell. The cardiac surgeon books for him to come in for his operation on the 1st of June and explains that he'll need to stay in hospital for several days afterwards to ensure that the operation has gone well, and support his recovery. Mr. Cohen prepares—it used to be the case that you would be admitted to the surgical ward the day before surgery and stay overnight, but again given the pressures on beds he is asked to come in early on the morning of the planned operation (nil by mouth from midnight etc.). The operation goes swimmingly, and he stays on the cardiothoracic ward for several days to make sure that he doesn't develop an infection, bleeding or some other recognised complication of surgery. On day three post-op there is a bit of a concern as he has a low blood pressure reading and then after some debate and discussion, he goes back to theatre for another look to ensure that everything is working and stitched together correctly. It turns out that he needs a bit of minor repair work but following this and a slightly extended Hospital stay he is released back onto the ward for a few days and then once well enough to go home, scheduled for an outpatient review in a month's time to see how he's getting on.

So those are two broad examples of the types of things that could bring you or one of your loved ones into Hospital. There are countless others and anything from a urinary tract infection to a broken hip will follow a similar pattern (admit, fix, assess response, discharge). Now irrespective of the clinical rationale for someone to be there, what else is involved in them inhabiting a hospital bed?

The resources and functions required include (but are not limited to); nurses and healthcare assistants to provide care, administer medications, and undertake the monitoring of physiological variables (pulse, temperature, blood pressure etc), the medical or surgical team to come and assess the patient every day, the Pharmacist review to check the medications, Physiotherapy to mobilise the patient, social services to sort out everything from carers to finances, Occupational therapy to make sure that the patient doesn't fall over again and will be safe at home, and lots of other allied health professional resources such as speech and language therapists and dieticians, plus theatre staff, porters, ward clerks and the facility sustaining costs of running a hospital, the electricity, the cleaners, structural maintenance and repair, PFI payments, the cost accountants, the list goes on because there is a lot that is bundled into the overall provision in-patient care, not just the upfront care from the Doctors and nurses. Estimates of the total costs of inhabiting a Hospital bed are around £483 per day in the UK, and $2883 in the US, but these figures are often disputed because it depends on what the patient is actually having done to them and the correct costing methodology being used [1, 2]. It's difficult to calculate the true direct and indirect costs of an average stay per patient (not only are the overheads of running a hospital significant, the electricity bill of a medium sized district general hospital for example are in the region of £2–3 million per year, but also medical teams are not very good at completing their discharge summaries to record events and interventions, which are used as the basis of the clinical codes that are used to bill the payor—the local clinical commissioning group, integrated health board or insurer).

There are two major aspects that could be altered to improve on this situation. Firstly, the patient experience is not ideal. Lying in an uncomfortable bed for days on end, on a noisy ward with unpleasant food, feeling vulnerable and exposed, is not conducive to wellbeing and recovery. Not forgetting that in-patient stays are potentially unsafe, with up to 10% of people admitted to hospitals experiencing some form of medical error.

Secondly, as with any service improvement imperative, is there any way that such high costs could be reduced—what are the ways to cut down on both the hotel elements for those patients not having much actively done for them and the blocking of beds for other needy recipients? In response to these concerns, wouldn't it much nicer, convenient, dignified and also cost-effective, to allow people to recover in their own homes, in their own beds?[1,2]

The factors described above have given rise to the necessary concept of the 'virtual ward', an alternative to in-patient bedded care, which is broadly speaking, a way of using technology to support patients requiring medical oversight (summarised in Fig. 3.2). Patients can be monitored on a semi- or completely remote basis and are looked after from afar. This is usually under the auspices of a secondary care team, who maintain responsibility for them and through the use of remote monitoring equipment and telehealth can review 'stable' patients either as a way of keeping them out of hospital (admission avoidance) or as a means of enabling earlier discharge whilst they wait for them to get better [4]. This is sometimes known as 'Hospital at Home' and the current definition from FutureNHS is that a virtual ward 'supports a person who would otherwise be in a secondary care bed' [5]. Just as in hospital, people on a

---

[1] Anecdotally people who smoke appear to mobilise (i.e. get up and start moving out of bed) after surgery much sooner than their non-smoking counterparts.

[2] According to the US Patient Safety Network, studies have consistently found that 10–12% of patients experience harm while hospitalised, with approximately half of these events being considered preventable [3].

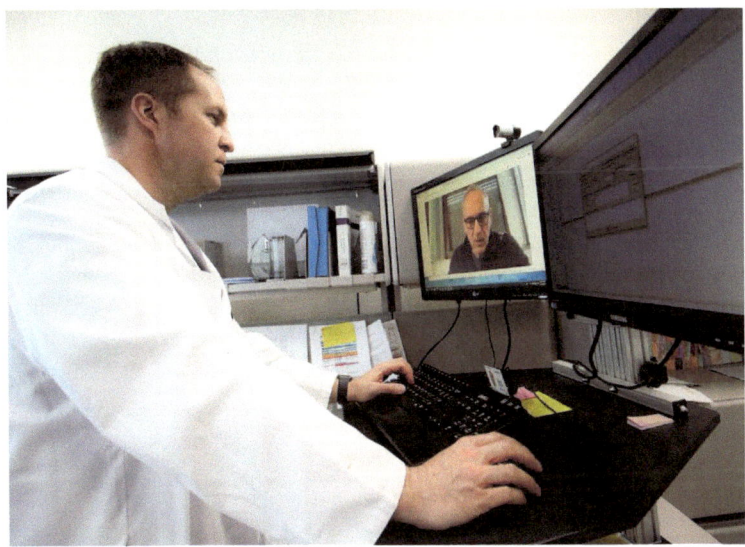

Fig. 3.2 Clinician reviewing a patient at home allocated to a virtual ward. Image Source: Defense Visual Information Distribution Service. Photo: Marcy Sanchez (unmodified from https://www. dvidshub.net/image/6182006/virtual-health-bridges-gap-patient-care-during-covid-operations) Commercial use authorised by DVIDS. The appearance of U.S. Department of Defense (DoD) visual information does not imply or constitute DoD endorsement

virtual ward are cared for by a multidisciplinary team who can provide a range of care interventions, tests and treatments. This could include blood tests, prescribing medication or administering fluids through an intravenous drip.

Box 3.1 Summary of the Components of Virtual Wards
What are Virtual Wards?

- Virtual wards support patients, who would otherwise be in hospital, to get the acute care, remote monitoring and treatment they need in their own home, including care homes and nursing homes.
- Virtual wards are suitable for a range of conditions which can be safely and effectively managed and monitored at home. Many local areas have developed or are developing virtual wards for a range of people including those with respiratory problems, heart failure or acute exacerbations of a frailty related condition.
- Patients are reviewed daily by the clinical team and the 'ward round' may involve a home visit or take place through telemedicine technologies. Many virtual wards use technology like apps, wearables and other medical devices enabling clinical staff to easily check in and monitor the person's recovery.

- Remote monitoring equipment and sensors gather patient data (e.g. images, symptoms, physiological observations) to give clinicians information that would normally only be obtainable in a face to face assessment, to improve clinical decision making, provide reassurance, and enable the early detection of deterioration. This may include solutions that are enabled by digital technology e.g. wearable devices.
- Virtual wards enable the management of avoidable admissions into hospital, or support early discharge out of hospital. They are seen as a safe and efficient alternative to in-patient bedded care across a wide range of scenarios.

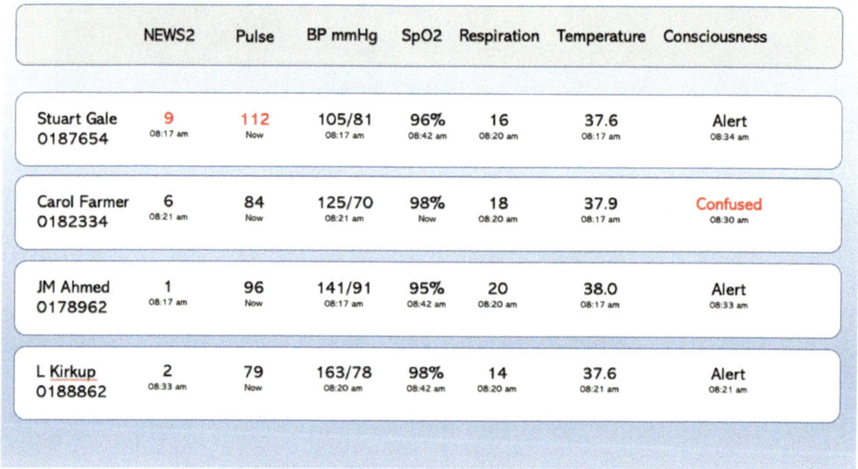

	NEWS2	Pulse	BP mmHg	SpO2	Respiration	Temperature	Consciousness
Stuart Gale 0187654	9 08:17 am	112 Now	105/81 08:17 am	96% 08:42 am	16 08:20 am	37.6 08:17 am	Alert 08:34 am
Carol Farmer 0182334	6 08:21 am	84 Now	125/70 08:21 am	98% Now	18 08:20 am	37.9 08:17 am	Confused 08:30 am
JM Ahmed 0178962	1 08:17 am	96 Now	141/91 08:17 am	95% 08:42 am	20 08:20 am	38.0 08:17 am	Alert 08:33 am
L Kirkup 0188862	2 08:33 am	79 Now	163/78 08:20 am	98% 08:42 am	14 08:20 am	37.6 08:21 am	Alert 08:21 am

Fig. 3.3 Example of a virtual ward dashboard

Patients on a virtual ward are reviewed regularly (usually daily) by a senior practitioner or a primary care Doctor via some form of technology enabled platform, who can assess their condition, review their treatment plan and solve any problems as they go (Fig. 3.3). If there is a clinical concern or the patient's condition is worsening, then there is generally a low threshold for escalating their care and bringing them back into a physical Hospital setting.

Virtual wards have become far more popular in recent years due to two main drivers, the COVID pandemic (forcing a re-evaluation of how we can deliver care in a world of limited bed capacity and the need to isolate and distance patients) and significant developments in the power and availability of digital monitoring technologies. Health services are increasingly introducing virtual wards for a variety of reasons, for example, for monitoring patients with respiratory infections or looking after elderly patients with frailty (a modern version of 'Hospital at Home'). This is facilitated by a variety of technological solutions including remote monitoring apps, pulse oximeters (to measure patient's levels of oxygen saturation), wearable sensors for heart rate and

MILD	**Low complexity** **COVID +** **Self caring** **No existing medical** **conditions**	**Referral threshold:** **Oxygen saturations > 95%** **Respiratory rate < 20** **New confusion** **NEWS2 score 0-2**	**Level of care:** **Pulse oximetry**
MODERATE	**Moderate complexity** **COVID +** **Underlying health** **conditions**	**Referral threshold:** **Oxygen sats 93-94%** **Respiratory rate 21-24** **New confusion** **NEWS2 score 3-4**	**Level of care:** **Oral antibiotics** **Inhalers** **Chest physiotherapy**
SEVERE	**High complexity** **COVID +** **Underlying health** **conditions**	**Referral threshold:** **Oxygen saturations < 92%** **Respiratory rate > 25** **New confusion** **NEWS2 score > 5**	**Level of care:** **IV antibiotics** **Steroids** **Nebulisers** **Oxygen therapy**
PALLIATIVE	**Moribunnd** **COVID +** **Families can be supported**	**Non-responsive / unlikely** **to respond to treatment /** **inappropriate to escalate** **care**	**Level of care:** **IV antibiotics** **Steroids** **Oxygen therapy** **Medication via pump**

Fig. 3.4 Suggested referral pathways and criteria for a Covid virtual ward

blood pressure, thermometers, motion detectors etc. plus, a combination of face-to-face care, such as district nurses and home visiting allied health professionals and remote communications, which could be phone, video or text based. Clinical teams see individual patient measurements for the cohort of patients they are responsible for, via some form of dashboard as above. The software that is used to facilitate virtual ward care is designed to alert the health care professionals when a patient's variables (such as their pulse rate or blood pressure) move outside of safe parameters, and then allows them to initiate any necessary actions (see Fig. 3.4). If the patient is deteriorating significantly then they can be whisked back into secondary care for review.

The use cases in practice typically tend to be for elderly and frail patients, those with several medical conditions such as heart failure, diabetes and COPD—both when those illnesses deteriorate, and when they have an acute medical problem such as an infective illness. Additionally, post-operative recovery and end of life care are good examples of where virtual ward care becomes very useful. The latter being relevant in an age where the majority of people would prefer to die at home in their own bed, rather than being stuck in a Hospital.

By providing healthcare professionals with the technology and tools to monitor qualifying patients at home, the aim is to reduce acute bed pressures and enable patients with less serious health needs to recover at home. "*It's a really exciting shift of patient management*," says Louise Hough, director of customer operations at Current Health. "*I think patients will always prefer to be in their own home, in their own bed, with their own family. They eat better, they sleep better, and they recover faster*" [6]. There are also—potentially—sizeable cost-savings to be had. One case study at Croydon Health Services NHS Trust found that virtual wards led to savings of over £742 per patient compared to a control group, with readmissions and hospital admissions post-discharge at 12% and 9%, respectively.

"Over that 17-month period they (the trust) had saved 4,642 bed days and a 70% reduction in patient readmissions, which I think is a staggering outcome," says Hough. Patient feedback survey scores were largely very positive, with over 87% of patients giving positive agreement with each statement given in the questionnaire. The areas patients were most positive about was the ease of learning to use the kit (89%) and the fact it was simple and easy to understand (89%). Alan Payne, group product and engineering director at Access Group refutes the idea that older patients might not be able to effectively use the technology needed to be monitored or to self-monitor at home. *"From all the virtual ward case studies happening across the country, it's clear that patients of all ages are open to being on a virtual ward and that using technology isn't holding them back"* [7].

The COVID-19 crisis provided an opportunity for specialist respiratory services to take on more patient care outside of the Hospital setting. One of the key aspects of COVID infection is the lengthy time it can take for an individual's lungs to recover to normal function. Patients can be dependent on receiving additional oxygen to help them breathe normally and usually this needs to be delivered in a hospital setting, with the correct facilities and monitoring set up (primarily in the form of an oxygen saturation monitor or pulse oximeter—one of those clever probes that clips to your finger, shining a strong light through the tissues to measure the amount of oxygen in the blood stream—which is a proxy measure of lung efficiency). There have traditionally been 'oximetry at home' programmes in which patients with chronic respiratory conditions on long term oxygen therapy are provided with their own pulse oximeters and are 'kept an eye on' by primary care. However, the volume and complexity of patients recovering from COVID-19 forced a switch to the secondary care sector to take on the monitoring and supervision of such patients in COVID virtual wards (see Fig. 3.5). This model (as exemplified by the award-winning chest team at Watford General Hospital led by Matthew Knight and Andy Barlow) facilitates earlier supported Hospital discharge (i.e. patients don't have to wait days or weeks in Hospital for their oxygen demands to return to normal) because patients are contacted daily as they would be on a regular hospital ward round by a specialist and through the use of remote monitoring, any deterioration in the patient's condition can be identified and their treatment escalated or a return to hospital triggered [8].

"The ultimate aim was to prevent hospital admission and facilitate early discharge, by providing specialist remote care to patients seven days per week at home. For this we needed data, provided remotely; data on patient's oxygen levels, pulse, respiratory rate, blood pressure and temperature as well as their symptoms"—says Matt Knight.

"Having patient data such as oxygen saturation readings, heart rate and temperature and symptoms in a structured and objective way meant we were able to double the number of patients we would care for simultaneously. At one point in wave 2 our virtual ward was vital for simultaneously caring for over 400 patients. The virtual ward allowed clinicians to work quickly through large amounts of patient collected data allowing me and my team to identify and focus on the 8.4% of patients who needed to be re-admitted. In some cases we were able to identify deteriorating patients long before they themselves presented these symptoms, undoubtedly saving lives".

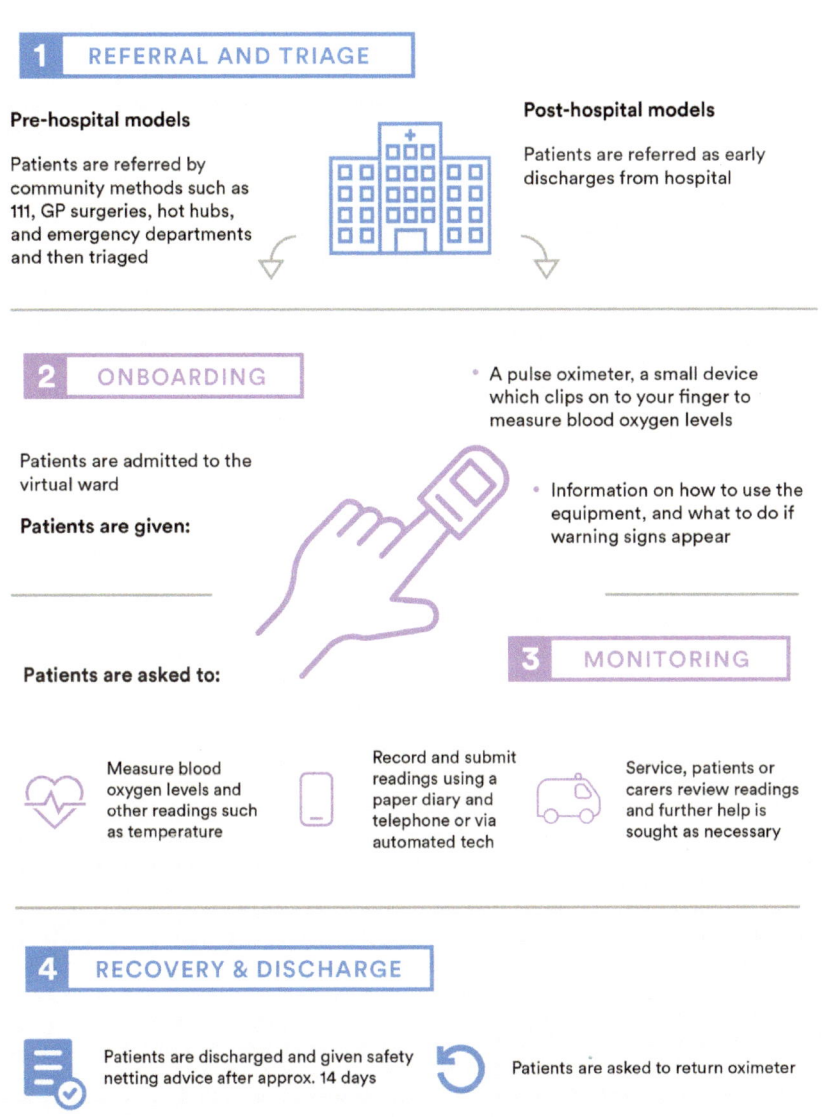

Fig. 3.5 Virtual ward care pathway. Image Source: Nuffield Trust, used with permission (https://www.nuffieldtrust.org.uk/resource/virtual-wards-and-covid-19-an-explainer). Originally produced by NIHR RSET (Rapid Service Evaluation Team), a partnership between the Nuffield Trust and University College London

In terms of outcomes, it was found that overall, less time was spent on each patient per day (due to a more focussed data review), an average of 3 minutes less, which when compounded, amounts to significant productivity gains. The re-admission rate (patients having to go back into Hospital) was much lower than normal (this perhaps relates to the pressures of getting patients out of hospital as quickly as possible) when compared to usual physical Hospital admission activity. Ninety-five percent of patients found the associated app (Medopad) easy to use and 76% of patients when surveyed felt happy to use this form of care again. Patients felt that care via the app was *"quicker, more flexible and allowed for constant monitoring without having to be in Hospital"*. Patient testimonials were positive along the lines of *"It was an easy app to use, which allowed me to maintain daily contact with the nurses and Doctors. I always got a call back when unwell to review my condition which I found very containing during an anxiety provoking time"*.

This type of care has been expanded significantly and was recommended by the NHS for rollout back in January 2021 (see Fig. 3.5). Over 90% of hospital trusts are now providing some form of virtual ward programme. Dr. Matt Inada-Kim a Consultant in Acute Medicine and 'National clinical director for infection, anti-microbial resistance and deterioration' has said that *"This now provides a blueprint for such community based, personalised care for a whole host of other conditions such as asthma, diabetes, high blood pressure, heart failure and COPD"*.

The case has been demonstrated well for reactive medical care, but what about proactive hospital avoidance? Several studies have shown that a large number of hospital admissions are predictable and potentially avoidable. Penny is a 74-year-old lady who lives alone. She suffers with osteoporosis, diabetes and has become increasingly frail. Her long-suffering GP is worried about her falling over and breaking a hip. He even managed to convince Penny at one stage to wear hip protectors (but she found wearing them uncomfortable so gave up). Her diabetes has become more unstable recently as she sometimes forgets to take her medication. In the autumn, she developed a urinary tract infection and started to get seriously unwell, she tried to contact the out of hours GP and they said they would send someone around, but they were overwhelmed with other calls. Penny wasn't eating and drinking very much, her glucose levels were erratic, she became dehydrated and fell over in the bathroom managing to wedge herself sideways between the toilet and the radiator. Two days later when Penny's daughter came round to visit her she found Penny stuck on the bathroom floor, moaning in discomfort, in a pool of her own urine, with both pressure sores and a second degree burn on her back from the radiator. When the paramedics arrived, they found that not only was she grossly septic but also had a very low blood glucose level.

Case studies of successful virtual ward interventions include in the city of Hull (led by Dr. Anna Folwell and Dr. Dan Harman, both community geriatricians) where people with frailty related problems are identified by a health professional such as a primary care Doctor, District Nurse or a Paramedic and then pass them on to the local virtual ward team for remote assessment either over the phone or by video link to check their suitability (using locally agreed criteria) [9]. 'Admission' to the virtual ward system follows and remote testing, for example ECG's, point of care blood testing, bladder scans to check for urinary retention, can be performed in the home setting, followed by the use of remote monitoring systems. Regular check-ins (again either by phone or video, as well as by in-person visits from district nurses, health care assistants, physiotherapists, paramedics etc.) and the initiation of relevant treatment—intravenous antibiotics for example can be safely given in the community, under the supervision of the infectious diseases team from afar. There are multiple benefits to this approach, chiefly as already mentioned, is that it reduces the strain on the hospital system, and it empowers people to remain in their home environment. This understandably increases both patient and carer satisfaction and would suit the example above with Penny.

An example of private sector innovation is from Doccla, set up in 2019 by Dag Larsson and Martin Ratz to harness the rapid uptake of tele-medicine, a Swedish medtech organisation that can deliver the virtual ward model at pace and scale on behalf of clients. This involves providing the tech side of things, (a home monitoring pack including the specialist equipment and a patient app through which the patient can submit their measurements and symptoms) the facilities for clinician communication, (video calls and messaging) and clinician support where needed—rather than just being a tech enabler.

If identified as suitable for a virtual ward before they leave Hospital, patients are given training on how to use the equipment and instructions on how to set the monitoring devices up at home themselves. Along with this they're provided with helpline numbers both in the event of equipment problems but also for clinical support if they are worried or start to become more unwell. When the patient's virtual ward 'stay' comes to an end all the monitoring kit is returned.

A rapid evaluation run by the Kent, Surrey and Sussex academic health science network and the Office for Life Sciences, of the Northampton virtual ward set up (facilitated by Doccla) showed that there was a shorter average length of stay for virtual ward patients and that this would have brought about significant cost savings in terms of reduced nursing costs (higher ratio of nurses per patients) and freed up capacity in the local acute setting [10]. They also found high levels of patient compliance which was likely contributed to by daily/chasing telephone calls from healthcare staff. Surveys showed that patient interactions with staff were an important factor in their recovery. Patient satisfaction levels were high and anecdotal reports suggest that the virtual ward approach helps to reduce anxiety and provide reassurance, *"That feeling of knowing that someone is keeping an eye on things for you"*. They also showed that staff satisfaction was high and because of the use of tech it enables healthcare staff who were shielding to continue to play a part in health care delivery. According to Fiona McCann one of the Respiratory Consultants from Northampton working with Doccla *"The service has exceeded all expectations, has truly thrived and has achieved excellence. Clients have embraced it. They love it, use it, and want it to continue"*, which seems like high praise indeed.

Internationally, countries in Sub-saharan Africa are also able to demonstrate the utility and effectiveness of the virtual ward concept. One interesting clinical practice review from The Gambia showed that the set-up of a virtual ward was possible even in a very overstretched health service (see Fig. 3.6). Dr. Ogehenebrume Wariri and his team from the London School of Hygiene and Tropical Medicine in Banjul, the capital of The Gambia, set up a virtual ward in their biomedical research facility [11]. They showed how they managed to assemble a muti-disciplinary team, create clear operating protocols and use telemedicine (including the use of closed

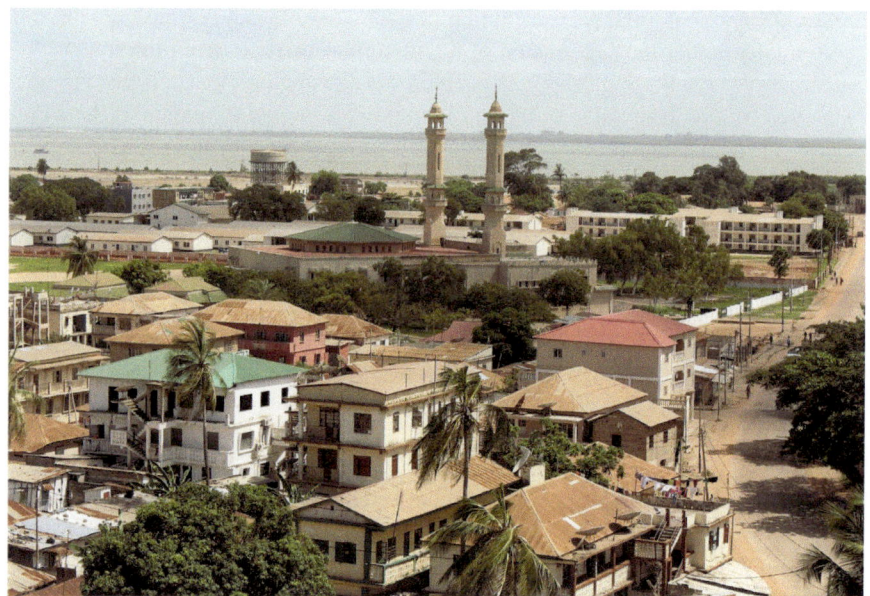

Fig. 3.6 Banjul, capital of The Gambia. Image source: Pixabay. Credit Issac Turay (https://pixabay.com/photos/cityscape-banjul-africa-gambia-2313618/). Reproduced with kind permission under the Pixabay content licence (https://pixabay.com/service/license-summary/)

WhatsApp groups for rapid communication) to consult with each other and patients, and to capture patient level data (using a digital thermometer and a pulse oximeter) to make the system a success and ensure that patients with infectious diseases could be looked after at home, with clear limits around escalating care if a patient's condition should get worse. This represents a prime opportunity for resource poor settings to take advantage of inexpensive technological solutions and overcome disparities in healthcare. However, the challenges of adequate staffing and limited budgets in such developing world settings are more prominent.

So far, the majority of virtual wards have been a combination of existing inpatient hospital facilities that extend their reach into the local community by having a number of virtual beds under their care umbrella—patients who would have otherwise come under their physical care. One amazing example of a complete shift to full virtual care is the Mercy Virtual Care Centre in The United States. This is a 54-million-dollar, 125,000 square foot facility in Chesterfield, Missouri, which has no patients or beds on site. It does have over 330 medical professionals based there who sit in front of a bank of computers in a clinical command centre. They are remotely taking care of patients in their homes and in beds across 38 hospitals in seven states (Arkansas, Kansas, Missouri, North Carolina, Oklahoma, Pennsylvania & South Carolina) so much further afield than in the local vicinity. Virtual care is delivered using highly sensitive two-way cameras, online-enabled instruments and real-time vital signs, allowing clinicians to "see" patients. A team of virtual hospitalists orders and reads tests, and nurses field questions about everything from nosebleeds to sinus infections. This centralised model demonstrates the power and reach of telemedicine's capability to work at scale and reduce costs. Mercy ultimately hopes to provide better care through more convenient and lower-cost locations. Program evaluations over the years show a 50% reduction in in-patient utilisation. There were 35% fewer days spent in the hospital system and there have been 60% fewer deaths from septic shock occurring in patients being treated remotely [12]. It makes sense that this model of care delivery will spread to other regions as a way of unifying and nationalising approaches to healthcare as well as more evenly distributing the workload.

Benefits and Limitations of Virtual Wards

The benefits of such approaches are clear to see, tracking symptoms and monitoring disease progression supports the proactive identification of patients at risk of deterioration. This can provide opportunities for earlier interventions. Virtual wards reduce the utilisation of scarce hospital resources down to the essential minimum required, this is better value for money and allows patients to recover in the comfort and safety of their own home and this is all facilitated by modern digital healthcare tech—which when mediated by safe and sensible clinical guidelines allows an alternative to traditional lengthy in-patient stays and reduces pressures on beds for those who truly need them.

There are obvious limits to these type of scenarios—you wouldn't want a septic, immobile individual at home by themselves being looked after virtually—but the use case for a large number of patients is clear and this viable alternative is welcome, especially when we can predict with mournful regularity the news headlines about the winter bed pressures and bed blockers affecting Hospitals every year.

There is strong support and interest in virtual wards because of the multiple benefits that they provide, and this is backed by an increasing evidence base. Patient feedback is positive, it empowers patient choice and independence. They reduce emergency hospital admissions because patients already have a care infrastructure in place and access to a multi-disciplinary team. They allow better utilisation of resources, especially when there are clear entry and exit criteria. The release of in-patient hospital beds has a major impact on the whole system. There is also some evidence to show that the use of virtual wards helps to improve staff experience. Enabling staff to undertake a mixture of blended remote and in-person care adds variety and reduces stress. Additionally, it allows those staff members unable to take direct clinical interactions (those who are shielding or burnt out) to continue to provide care.

Disadvantages of a virtual ward system of care are humanitarian (lonely, anxious patients being 'left alone' at their time of greatest need and often subtle signs of deterioration can't be spotted by a machine), economic (the evidence on cost savings is not fully there yet) and the overreliance on tech (leading to both risks of technical failure and also potential discrimination based on differing access requirements such as phone and broadband coverage—the 'digitally excluded' population). There are challenges in the collection of accurate data, with such rapid mobilisation there have been concerns about the lack of an adequate governance structure (who does what and what are the thresholds of concern, have all the risks been countered?). Might virtual wards become a dumping ground for hospitals to expedite people out of hospital too soon? There are also multiple ethical and legal issues such as liability and the protection of patient data.

Plus, there are concerns from some less than enthusiastic healthcare professionals, *"Some patients were recording worrying symptoms but when you spoke to on the phone, they were fine. The app created more calls and work"*. There is a concern about the frequent alerts and notifications both real and the false positives that happen with such systems. Clinicians (especially nursing staff) might be expected to increase their patient care workloads with no change in job plans or pay as there is an opinion that looking after virtual patients is 'easier and less intense' and because much of it can be automated, doesn't require the healthcare professional to do much. Interestingly the virtual ward concept does not appear to have taken off significantly in the United States and this might be for a variety of reasons such as cultural challenges (patients and Doctors disliking the idea of care being delivered remotely), concerns over litigation, lack of reimbursement from insurance companies and competition from traditional providers concerned about their market share.

The drive to generate supportive evidence has come from the team at Health Innovation Manchester who looked at key markers such as clinical outcomes, rates of patient death and numbers of readmissions to Hospital across several randomised controlled trials (the best format for a clinical study). They reviewed the available information and concluded that for these variables there is 'low to moderate' certainty evidence that patients treated in virtual ward settings they did as good or better than comparable Hospital in-patients. It's been highlighted that it is difficult to interpret the cost savings of such models in the studies undertaken so far (with many overestimating the potential savings) and this is unfortunate as cost-effectiveness is going to be one of the biggest motivators to take things forwards. It is also encouraging to see that the evidence supports that the greatest facilitators of successful virtual ward care include; patient acceptance, strong communication and organisational structures, coordinated multi-disciplinary teams and continuity of care. This means that this type of care delivery is not something that can be quickly and cheaply cobbled together. It has to be structured and supported more widely in order to work well.

From the literature and experience it appears that the main success factors for virtual wards are;

- Organisational factors (good set up and communication, access to the right level of clinical support and escalation when needed).
- Selection of the right patient groups who would derive most benefit (those who need time limited interventions with clear admission and discharge criteria).
- Patient centric design (acceptance, appropriateness, sensitivity, digital inclusion).
- Making life easy for clinicians (removing barriers to their work to allow them to focus on key clinical activities and decision making).

The NHS has been quick to see the value of such an approach and in their 2022–23 operational and planning guidance state that health systems should be aiming to deliver virtual ward capacity equivalent to 50 virtual ward beds per 100,000 population. This comes with additional central funding in order to provide support (£200 million funding has been made available from the Service Development Fund to support this initiative).

The ambition is ultimately to utilise virtual wards to increase overall acute bed capacity, using this resource safely and wisely (in order to avoid it becoming a dumping ground for chronic care patients) whilst exploiting remote monitoring technologies and digital platforms to deliver cost effective care. On several metrics this has already been successful. What is clear is that the cost modelling needs to be accurately done to ensure that its favourable to the existing model of in-patient care and that virtual hospital beds don't get co-opted into something that they are not suitable for.

The future for virtual wards is promising, with continued growth and evolution expected to transform the healthcare landscape in several ways:

1. **Wider Adoption:** virtual wards are likely to be more widely adopted by healthcare systems worldwide. As the benefits of virtual care become increasingly evident, more hospitals and healthcare providers are likely to implement virtual ward models to extend their reach and improve patient care for suitable individuals.
2. **Integration of Advanced Technologies:** as we gather more and more data on patients receiving virtual care, artificial intelligence (AI), machine learning (ML), and data analytics will play a crucial role in patient risk prediction, personalised treatment plans, and continuous monitoring of health metrics, leading to the development of increasingly smart clinical decision support tools.
3. **Wearable and IoT Integration:** wearable devices and the Internet of Things (IoT) will become integral to virtual ward setups. Patients will use these devices to monitor their vital signs, activity levels, and health data, providing real-time information to healthcare providers. The type and level of sophistication of such technologies is growing rapidly.
4. **Remote Surgical Consultations:** virtual wards will enable remote surgical consultations and post-operative care, reducing the need for in-person visits and hospital stays. This will be especially valuable for patients in remote areas or those with limited mobility.
5. **Mental Health Support:** the future of virtual wards will emphasise mental health support and teletherapy, for which there is a current huge demand. As the importance of mental health care continues to grow, virtual ward models will incorporate mental health services, peer support and counselling.
6. **Global Reach:** virtual wards will facilitate cross-border healthcare delivery, allowing patients to access specialised care from providers in different countries. International collaboration in healthcare will become more accessible and efficient.

7. **Predictive and Preventive Care:** there will increasingly be a focus on predictive and preventive care. AI algorithms will identify patients at risk for certain conditions and initiate interventions before health problems worsen.

8. **Enhanced Interoperability:** improved interoperability between virtual ward systems and different healthcare platforms will facilitate seamless information exchange between providers, laboratories, and pharmacies, leading to more coordinated and patient-centric care.

9. **Regulatory Advances:** regulatory bodies will play a vital role in shaping the future of virtual wards. New guidelines and regulations will likely be developed to ensure patient safety, privacy, information governance and the quality of virtual care services.

10. **Cost-Efficiency:** this model of care will hopefully continue to contribute to cost savings for healthcare systems. By reducing hospital admissions and readmissions, virtual care can alleviate the financial burden on healthcare providers and patients alike.

11. **Patient Empowerment:** virtual wards will arguably empower patients to take a more active role in their own health management. Patients will have access to their health data, allowing them to make informed decisions and collaborate with their care teams and understand their own condition and progress. Depending on their suitability, patients may pro-actively elect to receive virtual ward care.

12. **Environmental Sustainability:** the digital nature of virtual wards aligns with the growing emphasis on environmental sustainability in healthcare. Reduced physical visits and energy-efficient technology, reduced travel emissions and less burden on the Hospital estate, can contribute to a more sustainable healthcare system.

Overall, the future of virtual wards lies in their ability to provide accessible, personalised, and proactive healthcare that has a good evidence base with regards to improved patient outcomes, reduced costs, and extends the reach of medical expertise. As technology continues to advance, virtual wards will become an essential component of modern healthcare, supporting a patient-centric and data-driven approach to well-being.

Summary

Virtual wards therefore seem to be a smart solution to solving the chronic problems of bed blockade and insufficient capacity that we have been familiar with for many years. The perfect storm of opportunity, health service pressures and the COVID-19 pandemic collided at a time when software and technology (and most importantly—the necessary mindset change) were present to allow the creation and honing of new ways of delivering 'hospital standard care' outside of the traditional hospital setting.

This is exciting because it in principle allows healthcare professionals to work in new ways, to look after more patients more efficiently and overcome the need for physical hospital beds. Patients are also generally in favour too because admission to hospital can be a daunting and stressful experience. The issues of safety still need to be high on the agenda, especially because we are still in the early days of using remote monitoring technologies—it will only take a few examples of deleterious outcomes (alerts being ignored, equipment failing, patient's blowing up their own oxygen supplies, monitors not identifying a moribund patient) to throw a spanner in the virtual works. As such, clear entry and exit criteria, and safety monitoring guidelines need to be in place both for the technical and clinical aspects of care and the role of the 'clinical safety officer' will be paramount to ensure that virtual ward systems of care are safe and reliable. In reality this should be balanced with the fact that the risk of any type of medical error affecting an in-patient hospital stay can be high so it will be interesting to see over time what the rate of significant events and calamities relating to virtual ward care will be (data collection is key). Finally, the main factor determining the success of virtual ward models is going to come down to cost, will early discharge and hospital avoidance schemes reap the financial benefits that are so desperately needed? Only time will tell.

References

1. Typical US hospital stay costs 384 hours of work with average earnings. Value Penguin. https://www.valuepenguin.com/hospital-bill-costs-study#:~:text=typical%20hospital%20stay.-,The%20average%20per%2Dday%20hospital%20cost%20is%20%242%2C883%2C%20but%20the,cost%20was%20%241%2C102%20a%20day. Accessed 29 Oct 2023.
2. Nowpatient. How much do I cost the NHS? https://nowpatient.com/health-news/how-much-do-i-cost-the-nhs. Accessed 29 Oct 23.
3. Patient Safety Network. Adverse events, near misses, and errors. 2019. https://psnet.ahrq.gov/primer/adverse-events-near-misses-and-errors. Accessed 28 Oct 2023.
4. Arsenault-Lapierre G, Henein M, Gaid D, Le Berre M, Gore G, Vedel I. Hospital-at-home interventions vs in-hospital stay for patients with chronic disease who present to the emergency department: a systematic review and meta-analysis. JAMA Netw Open. 2021;4(6):e2111568. https://doi.org/10.1001/jamanetworkopen.2021.11568.
5. Health Innovation Manchester. Virtual wards and hospital at home. https://healthinnovation-manchester.com/our-work/virtual-wards-and-hospital-at-home/
6. Current Health. Rapid evaluation of the virtual ward at Croydon NHS. https://www.curren-thealth.com/insights/guides/rapid-evaluation-of-the-virtual-ward-at-croydon-nhs/
7. Hughes O. Special report: virtual care. Digital Health 2023. https://www.digitalhealth.net/2023/10/special-report-virtual-care-2/
8. Tech-enabled virtual wards: relieving pressure on the NHS while caring for patients at home. https://transform.england.nhs.uk/key-tools-and-info/data-saves-lives/improving-individual-care-and-patient-safety/virtual-wards-relieving-pressure-on-the-nhs-while-caring-for-patients-at-home/
9. NHS England. Supporting people living with frailty in Hull and East Riding. 2021. https://www.england.nhs.uk/virtual-wards/case-studies/case-study-supporting-people-living-with-frailty-in-hull-and-east-riding/

10. Northamptonshire Virtual Wards. Rapid evaluation—summary report. 2022. https://
    uploads-ssl.webflow.com/5e4bb3071e21af55553b2fcb/6283f478f0cea4ccd61b2aca_
    Northamptonshire%20Virtual%20Wards%20Rapid%20Evaluation%20Report%20NHSX.pdf
11. Wariri O, Okomo U, Cerami C. Establishing and operating a 'virtual ward' system to provide
    care for patients with COVID-19 at home: experience from The Gambia. BMJ Glob Health.
    2021;6:e005883.
12. Mercy Case Study. How Mercy built a technology-enhanced care management model to
    scale care management and increase patient engagement. https://f.hubspotusercontent10.net/
    hubfs/6835019/Mercy%20Case%20Study%202020-1.pdf

Further Reading

O'Malley E-J, Hansjee S, Abdel-Hadi B, Kendrick E, Lok S. A Covid-19 virtual ward
    model: a preliminary retrospective clinical evaluation from a UK District General
    Hospital. J Prim Care Community Health. 2022;13:21501319211066667. https://doi.
    org/10.1177/21501319211066667.

Chapter 4
The Virtual Clinic

Abstract The emergence of virtual out-patient services is transforming the way that patients access and experience medical care. It's important to explore this transformative shift, delving into the ground-breaking developments, challenges, and opportunities that have arisen with the integration of technology and new ways of working into out-patient care. The potential benefits of such approaches include increased access to care, reduced waiting times, improved patient outcomes and more cost-effective care delivery. The downsides relate to the need for a significant mindset change from Doctors, patients and Hospital managers and important issues such as data security, the need for an effective telehealth infrastructure, and problems around digital exclusion. This chapter explores the successes and lessons learned in the adoption of virtual out-patient services.

Keywords Out-patients · Virtual clinic · Virtual hospital · Remote care · Telemedicine · Tele-health · Elective care · Patient self-service · Empowerment · Patient engagement

The Out-Patient Service

'Out-patient' departments have existed as an appendage of Hospitals for as long one may care to remember. Their function being to see and treat people not sick enough to require an 'in-patient' stay. In his history of the Royal College of Physicians, Sir George Clark describes an embryonic form of out-patient clinic at the Hotel Dieu in Paris in the seventeenth century, '*Six Physicians were detailed for regular sessions on Wednesdays and Saturdays, advising the poor individually and consulting together when necessary....it was an innovation in that it did something for sufferers who would not have come into the Hospital wards*' [1].

Robert Bridges, working at Bart's Hospital in 1878 wrote how he personally had to filter over 30,000 patients per year, two thirds of them new patients, at an average rate of one every 88 s [2]. It has long been argued that overcrowding of out-patient departments and the hurry with which people are seen leads to mistakes and a poor quality of care. A production line approach to medicine which still exists in the present that arguably conflicts with the best values of health services.

Today we are in the situation where the vast majority of people with disease don't require Hospital admission (this is reserved for the most acutely unwell and gone are the days of the lying-in and convalescent Hospitals). They can be looked after by the booming industry that has become out-patient services and given the growing knowledge and complexity of modern medicine this becomes sub-divided into a multitude of medical and surgical sub-specialities (everything from Uro-Gynaecology to Audio-vestibular medicine). One of the most critical measures of the quality of a country's health care system is how long patients have to wait to access medical care (Fig. 4.1). Out-patient attendances and waiting lists for appointments are at an all-time high, over 7.8 million as of early 2024 in the UK and similarly high in countries across the developed world [3]. In a study of healthcare waiting times by country it was shown that in the US 27% of patients had to wait longer than 1 month on average to see a specialist, the figures for France, Germany and Canada were 36%, 25% and 61% respectively [4]. A report from the Australian Medical Association on the problem of 'the hidden waiting list', highlighted that in some areas of Australia waiting times were significant [5]. In Victoria, a patient will wait more than 900 days for an urgent neurosurgery appointment (target 30 days). In Queensland, a patient will wait more than 150 days for an urgent gastroenterology or rheumatology appointment (target 30 days). And for non-urgent

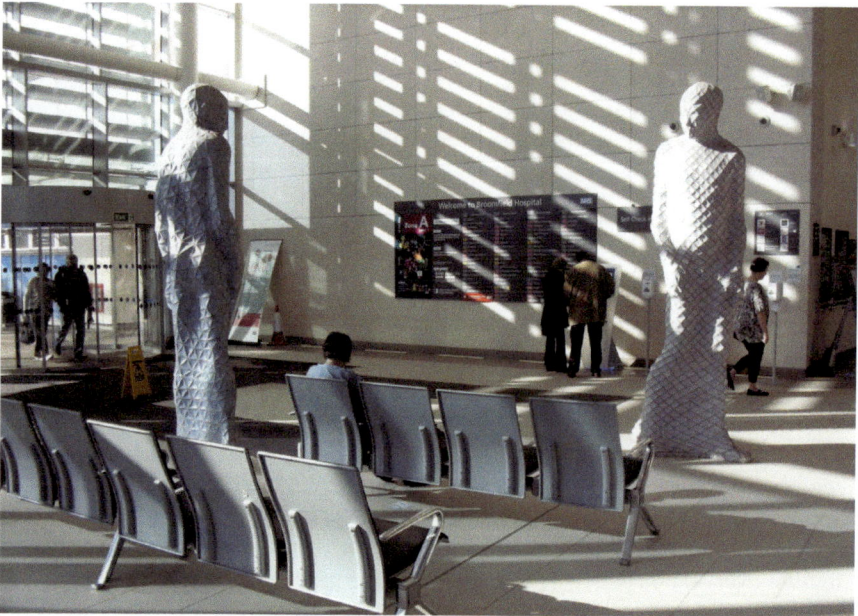

Fig. 4.1 A contemporary out-patient waiting room. Copyright Peter Stack and licensed for reuse under Creative Commons Licence attribution sharealike 2.0 generic. https://creativecommons.org/licenses/by-sa/2.0/ (Unmodified from Source: https://www.geograph.org.uk/photo/2816738)

appointments in Queensland and Victoria, waiting times for ophthalmology, ortho-paedics, and plastic/reconstructive appointments are all more than 700 days in both states (target 365 days).

This problem of high demand and long waits is contributed to by an ageing popu-lation and a rise in multi-morbidity and we're in a struggle to meet demand because of the residual impacts of COVID-19, limited clinical capacity and organisational barriers amongst many other factors. The NHS for example has a commitment for all newly referred patients to be seen by a specialist and treatment commenced within 18 weeks. This is an admirable target but achieving this is proving very dif-ficult. It is a *wicked* problem to solve, especially with the backlog of problems caused by the pandemic, mismanagement and political interference.

The Traditional Patient Journey

There is also the issue of how the out-patient process works. A patient with a head-ache or angina pains or dizzy spells cannot directly access a specialist Doctor such as a Neurologist or a Cardiologist. If something is persistent and problematic enough for them to need help, an individual (or their significant other) has to get an initial meeting with their primary care Doctor (the so-called gatekeepers of second-ary care). The primary care Doctors who are over worked and harried will attempt to sort out the medical problem, initiate some basic tests and the first line of man-agement in order to try and ameliorate things and send the patient on their way. For the vast majority of problems this tends to work very well as most conditions tend to self-limit and will respond to the ministrations of the busy Doctor. If the problem doesn't settle down or piques a certain level of severity, the primary care team needs to consider getting the specialist at the local hospital involved. They need to write a letter of referral to their Hospital counterpart to explain what's going on, and that they need them to be investigated and managed in the out-patient setting. However, there are several barriers and perverse incentives that may stymie this seemingly simple approach. Firstly, Hospitals are overloaded with referrals and often receive a significant number of sub-optimal requests where either the primary care Doctor has not covered all the basics that might be expected, they've got the wrong special-ity, they don't meet the right criteria for care, or the desired service is no longer provided. Secondly, the local health authorities or health insurers, who are desper-ately trying to balance their budgets, recognise that an excess of referrals into sec-ondary care from their primary care networks, is going to cost them money. Therefore, there is a tendency to throw a net around referrals, by either capping the number, penalising practices who refer 'too many' patients or intensely scrutinising each and every referral to make sure that it can be justified in terms of potential value. There are positives and negatives to these approaches and it's a frustration that primary care Doctors have to jump over multiple hurdles to get what they need for decent patient care.

The letter of referral then gets posted, faxed, or if you are lucky, emailed to the out-patient specialist (it may sit in an actual or electronic in-tray for some time) and is then briefly read by a busy Consultant to see whether it warrants an out-patient appointment to be greenlit or not. It then goes into another pile for booking and depending on how stretched the service is, it could sit there for several weeks or months before an appointment is tentatively booked for the patient. The appointment will then hopefully happen several months down the line and the patient will attend and finally get seen.

On the day of the first appointment, the patient takes the morning off work and makes the trek to the Hospital, finds a car parking space and takes out a small loan to pay for the ticket. They sit in the crowded waiting room of the out-patients department when they eventually find it (in the portacabin at the back of the Hospital) and after only a short delay get to see not the Consultant or the Attending Physician or Surgeon, but his junior (the Doctor in training) who explains that they need some more information about their medical history (called a clerking—because they don't have access to their full care record) and then they present the findings to the Consultant who will decide what happens next. The patient then answers a wide range of questions about their medical problem (in a fair amount of depth) to try and figure out what is going on. The trainee disappears next door to present their case to the busy senior Doctor who may or may not pop their head in to say hello to the patient, before dictating a course of action. This management plan generally involves organising a set of investigations to get to the bottom of their issues and allow the medical team to establish the diagnosis and an eventual treatment plan.

Several paper request forms are completed and signed for blood tests, urine analysis, radiology scans, stool tests (if you're lucky) and endoscopies as required. The patient is then sent away with instructions of variable quality about how to proceed and when to do what is needed. Because all these tests are done by different departments the patient may have to make several further trips to the Hospital to get them done ('Please could I arrange for the blood test on the same day that I'm coming in for my scan?', "No").

The results of the various diagnostic investigations will eventually trickle across the clinician's desk for them to review and sign off, and unless there is anything very worrying about them, nothing will be done straight away.

The patient will have been booked in for a follow up appointment a few months down the line and may even get to see the Consultant at that stage. They'll be asked how they are doing and discuss the test results that have come back. In some cases, not everything may have been completed. They could still on the waiting list for the definitive test e.g. a colonoscopy, and it's due in a month's time (or it was the wrong test that was ordered, or the test couldn't be completed on the day, or the registrar forgot to request contrast studies). This means that we have not yet established what is going on with the patient and the appointment was essentially wasted as this was the critical test. Nothing can be done yet in terms of initiating treatment. There will be a search for a clinic appointment straight after the colonoscopy, however there are no slots available in a month, so come back in a further 2 months' time to discuss the results.

At the end of this journey to diagnosis. The patient comes back to clinic, hopefully has their diagnosis established and explained, and treatment can finally be initiated. They have had to wait a considerable amount of time, experienced multiple pain points and inconveniences along the way, and have continued to suffer (experiencing the progression of their symptoms) all throughout this wait. They may continue to experience similar issues with waiting, communication failures and disorganisation as they remain in the Hospital system for follow up care and long-term management.

Is this the best system of care? Would you end up with such a process if you designed things from scratch today? One might argue that the concept of out-patients services is out-dated and no longer fit for purpose. The system is overwhelmed, inefficient, relies on primary care Doctors to do the right thing at the right time and to fill in the referral form in the correct way (otherwise it's back to square one). It doesn't seem to be a sustainable, working model as things are at the moment. There is a lot of wasted time and hoops to jump through. This is well recognised within the health service and by Governments. Recent research by the charity Engage Britain has discovered that 10% of adults in the UK have turned to independent or private healthcare providers in the year 2021–2022. Of those, two thirds did so because they were being subject to prolonged waiting list delays or just could not access treatment on the NHS [6]. Miriam Levin, health and care programme director at Engage Britain, said: *"While the NHS still unites many of us with a feeling of pride, it's clear more and more people feel forced to turn to private treatment. As people suffer through months of pain and discomfort after postponed appointments, or waste time and energy chasing up referrals, millions are feeling desperate enough to use savings or get into debt to help us get well"*.

The challenge is how can this system be transformed and modernised to enhance quality of care, reduce wait times and improve productivity?

Re-Imagining Out-Patient Services

Back in 2013, a young Gastroenterology doctor in training, named Bahman Shokouhi, working at the Whittington Hospital in North London was slogging his way through a busy clinic, seeing one patient after another in quick succession. The process is familiar to all those exposed to the busy world of out-patients. You work your way through a list of new and follow up patients, they are supposed to be allocated to set time slots, but clinics never run to time and it's a struggle to give people the time and attention that they deserve. Bahman picked up a new set of notes and called a patient in from the waiting room. Before she had even got to the consulting room door, he had read the referral letter and realised that she did not need to be there, that this was going to be a wasted appointment and this eventuality could have been headed off several weeks, if not months before.

The patient had a simple problem, one that required a straightforward test that could have been easily completed at the beginning of their referral journey, the result could have been reviewed and a care plan and advice provided without her ever having to see a specialist or wait the 8 months it took to get a physical out-patient appointment. This is because the system was not set up or incentivised to review people in advance or use some form of remote review in order to expedite patient care. It was still based on the system of people requiring a referral as ticket of valid entry to the specialist system, followed by a prolonged wait to get a 15 min appointment with a specialist.

Bahman, rather than pointlessly bemoaning the situation, decided to do something about it. He realised that if primary care referrals could be dealt with more directly, at the point of origin (obviating a waiting list system) then you could work out who really needed specialist care in person, what blood tests and scans would be useful to do straight away, based on the referral information, what could be dealt with by simple advice and guidance and in certain cases, those people who sounded really sick and needed to come to clinic could attend much sooner. By focussing on delivering attentive care early on, patients could be worked up before they got to clinic, which meant that they wouldn't have a meaningless and inefficient wait. With some technical support he set up an online platform to allow the receipt of primary care referrals (via email, rather than by letter!), allowing clinicians to log in remotely and review the cases and effectively run an asynchronous out-patient service. Thus, 'Medefer', was born. A virtual out-patient clinic. Doctors could review new referral information—immediately following a referral from primary care—they could decide on what to do next and initiate those steps that would have otherwise taken place in the out-patient clinic several months down the line. If there was not enough information about a patient's history, ('this patient has really bad indigestion, please review') then the Doctor or their junior could call them up and take their medical history over the phone. If a set of blood or stool tests were needed to guide decision making, then these could be ordered, and the patient could go off and get them directly. If it seemed like they had been referred to the wrong speciality (they may need to see an upper GI surgeon instead of a Gastroenterologist) then they could be diverted elsewhere in a timely fashion. In short, the majority of tasks that you might undertake on a first visit to a physical out-patient clinic, could be done well in advance and through remote means. The Consultant starts to put the pieces of the patient's jigsaw together well before seeing them. And in many cases, the patient never needs to physically attend at all.

The consequences of this are significant. At a stroke, it is possible to enhance patient care by doing all the necessary triage and work up tasks very quickly indeed right up front. The numbers of inappropriate or unnecessary referrals reaching outpatient clinics are dramatically reduced. For those that do need to attend in person, waiting list times are decreased and by the time they get there, they are more fully worked up, meaning that only the more complex patient cases are seen (the rest being safely dealt with by remote means). Most importantly patient care and safety are improved. It is more convenient and efficient for many patients not to have to come to clinic (taking time off work, getting to the hospital, finding parking, waiting for a long time for a rushed appointment etc.) and people are often pleasantly surprised by how quickly their case is reviewed and dealt with by a specialist. The

Medefer approach does not work for all patients and there are several exceptions, including those with suspected cancer, but on the whole, it works very well because it uses a simple paradigm shift to improve patient care by moving away from the traditional bricks and mortar approach and managing patients virtually. Ultimately the demand for out-patient services is cut down and principle of the model is that the waiting times for those that do need to attend in person are much swifter.

Over the past decade Medefer has scaled up significantly and has become an independent healthcare provider in its own right, using clinicians from not just across the country, but from around the world, to provide services. It is the first (and only) CQC registered virtual hospital service in the UK and has grown and diversified to cover multiple medical and surgical specialities, working with a variety of traditional providers across the UK and internationally, providing specialist care to regions that commonly have major waiting list problems or struggle to recruit enough clinicians to deal with local demands. It's clinical advisory board now includes such luminaries as Patricia Hewitt (the former secretary of state for Health and Sir Mike Richards the form Chief Inspector of Hospitals). The results reported by Medefer show the impact of introducing a virtual clinic service; the average time from initial patient referral to first Consultant review is only 18 h, in-person outpatient attendances can be reduced by up 70%, the average time required to clear a patient waiting list is 5 weeks per speciality and importantly, patient satisfaction levels are high at greater than 90% because of the speed, convenience, and quality of the model [7].

Examples of Virtual Clinics

A very similar model to Medefer, is provided by Xyla, whose service process is demonstrated in the flow chart below (Fig. 4.2).

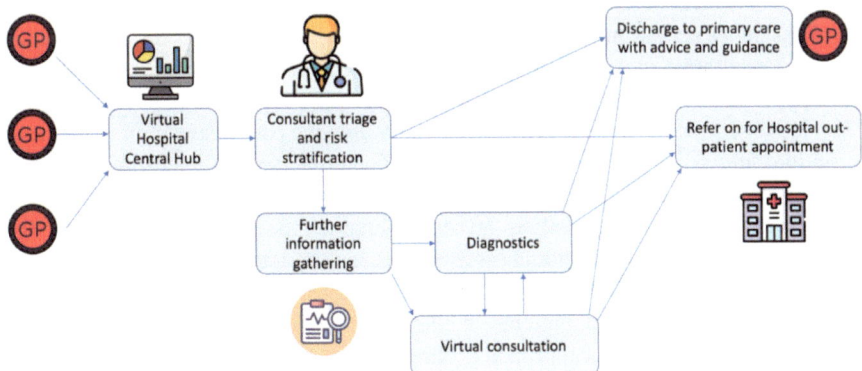

Fig. 4.2 Patient virtual management pathway

Results similarly show a reduction in the numbers of patients needing to physically attend out-patient clinics. Alongside this they also provide an advice and guidance network for primary care Doctors, through which specialist expertise can be tapped into without the need for a more formal (and costly) specialist referral.

The integrated care board in Frimley (southwest of London) used Xyla services for specialist Dermatology support when the routine waiting times for out-patient clinics ballooned in excess of 80 weeks. They were able to set up a system in which teledermatology (uploading of skin images onto a medical platform) could be used as a way of allowing remotely based Dermatologists to review photographs, eliminate the need for face-to-face appointments and get a much earlier specialist opinion and management plan. The outcomes of this project were encouraging, with a 40% reduction in 2 week wait referrals (for suspected skin cancer) going through to secondary care, and an overall diversion of 40% of referrals being able to be managed outside of the traditional clinic or referred back to primary care without the need for specialist intervention [8]. Dr. Rob Ellis, Consultant Dermatologist made clear his delight with this approach, *"I truly believe that Teledermatology provides the optimum model for dermatology services of the future. Initial assessment of referrals is made by Consultant Dermatologists, allowing early diagnosis and a bespoke pathway for every patient. The seamless integration with Primary Care means I can rapidly reassure patients with benign skin lesions or enable swift access to specific skin cancer services. Rashes receive optimum initial therapies within hours, rather than waiting months for appointments. It also fosters education and learning for GPs with immediate feedback on proposed diagnoses and management plans."*

Examples of virtual clinics from elsewhere in the world, include HelloHealth or the MyClevelandClinic app, which enables patients to remotely interact with their usual clinician via a smartphone or computer, and doxy.me which provides a telemedicine platform that healthcare providers (large or small) can white label and use to schedule and deliver virtual clinic appointments online and is used by organisations such as the Virginia Department of Health and Baton Rouge General. Arguably however, these US systems merely replicate the existing system online rather than being particularly innovative.

Both Xyla and Medefer demonstrate a type of clinic working somewhat different to what many people might generally consider a virtual clinic to be, i.e. an online video consultation in which a patient interacts with a Doctor much like they would in a physical setting. Whilst this does happen in an increasing number of out-patient services, these newer approaches actually uncouple the patient and clinician interaction into an *asynchronous* way of working. The clinician can undertake a desktop review of the patient's medical information and make diagnoses, investigation requests and management plans at times separate to direct patient interaction. Indeed, when patient contact and discussion is required, this could be scheduled by phone or video at a different time and utilise other care professionals, such as more junior Doctors, to take the patients' medical history or to relay the results of diagnostic investigations. This approach is based around enhancing the senior clinicians work to be more focussed and directed. If you can provide the essential information to a Doctor and remove the time wasted having to chase test results or gather data for themselves then you can facilitate significant productivity gains from this essential resource. If you want Doctors to function better, then you have to make things easier and more efficient for them.

Other ways of improving the out-patient journey can be considered in terms of optimising the pathway itself through the concept of clinical-digital transformation. Open Medical is a clinically led software company, founded by Dr. Harry Lykostratis, an Orthopaedic surgeon and software engineer. He has developed an entire platform, called Pathpoint, designed to improve the flow of patient care. Patient referrals are captured from multiple sources and the application expedites patient cases through the system, taking care of the administrative processes, helping to provide a holistic overview of patient care and standardising care delivery depending on the particular medical or surgical speciality. The outcome improvements that they've achieved by using this managed approach to patient care are exciting and include significant reductions (20%) in the time taken between injury and treatment for orthopaedic patients, a reduction in unnecessary appointments with 53% of referrals being triaged straight to the appropriate procedure, a 12% decrease in Hospital admissions and significant cost and efficiency savings realised in the Hospital services where this approach has been deployed [9].

Patient Self-Service

When it comes to reducing the burden of workload for the clinician, how about allowing the patient themselves to doing some of the work? You're probably very familiar with the scenario of having to provide your medical details repeatedly to your primary care Doctor, the nurse, the administrator, the specialist and so on, constantly thinking that there must be a better way of capturing and storing this data for ease of use. The traditional system that healthcare professionals use for exploring and recording your medical details is known as 'history taking' and follows a fairly standardised process of asking you about each of your presenting complaints in detail (how long have you had it for, where does it hurt, what makes things better or worse etc.). Learning these questions and knowing what to ask when is a key part of Doctors training. It's not particularly hard though and anyone with a script could run through it. The synthesis of the information gathered is the tricky part but the actual data gathering is something that could be done through a self-completed form or template. Medefer have actually been trialling such a system, known as 'preDoc' which provides a series of prompts and questions for patients to fill in themselves online and then structures the responses into a classic clinical type narrative, populated with your personal information. Your inputs from questions related to headache symptoms can then be assembled for the reviewing clinician into a digestible format, for example, '*Miss **Davison**, a **42** year old **Engineer**, with a past medical history of **Asthma**, describes a **6 month** history of progressively worsening **frontal headaches**. She describes these as **burning in nature** and have a severity of **7 out of 10***', and so on. Such an approach saves a great deal of clinical time and empowers patients to provide their own unbiased version of events. By standardising the question set it means that variations in care are ironed out. Specifically, 'red flag' symptoms, (those associated with potential life-threatening conditions such as cancer) won't be missed or forgotten. Over time, such systems can learn from the inputs and provide a useful substrate for clinical decision support tools and present investigation and treatment options to Doctors who can then review and approve. For example, organisations such as Infermedica are applying AI and ML to learn from patient inputs in order to develop likely diagnosis lists and suggested management plans before a clinician is even involved.

Pros and Cons

The advantages of virtual clinics include—the costs and convenience factors—patients and their families/carers not having to travel to the Hospital or take time off school or work, there is greater environmental sustainability because of the associated reduction in carbon emissions (and importantly easier car parking for the rest of us). Attendance at clinic appointments may be better than with an in-person appointment and they can be easier to reschedule, leading to a reduction in 'Did-Not-Attend' rates. There will also be fewer patients waiting in the normal clinic spaces which will help to reduce the spread of infectious illnesses (Fig. 4.3). Virtual clinics allow the utilisation of a far larger pool of clinicians given that they can access platforms and manage patients from virtually anywhere and across more timeframes, this helps to tackle the regional variations in demand and capacity and the restrictive 9–5 weekday clinic opening times. It also leads to greater clinician

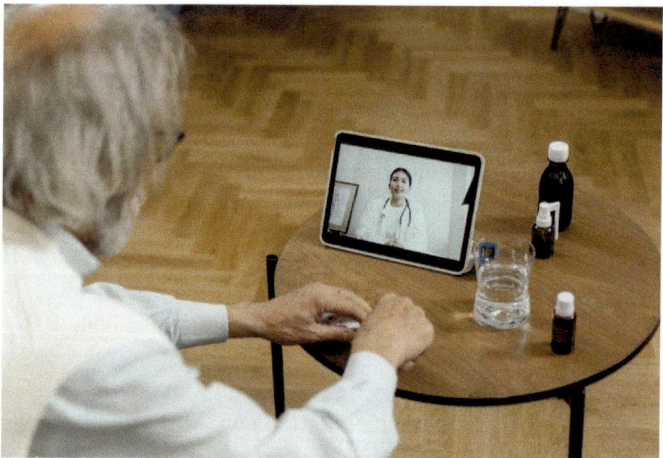

Fig. 4.3 A remote Doctor video consultation. Credit: Tima Miroshnichenko. Reproduced under permission from Pexels. (Unmodified from Source: https://www.pexels.com/photo/a-doctor-doing-an-online-consultation-8376177/)

satisfaction because they know that time is being used more effectively and this overcomes many of the frustrations faced by healthcare professionals [10].

Potential disadvantages may include the challenges of setting up the right digital infrastructure and interoperability of different systems to enable such a system to work. Remotely requesting an investigation to take place in Hull when you're based in Aberdeen may prove technically difficult at first. Digital exclusion has been cited as one of the drawbacks if patients do not have access or the competence to use online systems, however, with models such as those rolled out by Medefer, on the patient side, no specific tech is needed, and the system can function effectively on the basis of physical letters and telephone calls. More philosophically, patients may feel that they are being dealt with in a more transactional manner and that not being seen face to face can diminish the quality of care that they receive. This is true to a certain extent; patients might be seen as a set of problems to be fixed on a never ending production line. Whilst virtual triage, review and management works well for a great many conditions and is very convenient for busy patients, it's important to never underestimate the human aspects of clinical care delivery and always allow for an opt-out approach so that patients who want that extra dimension of care can always access the traditional model and develop the Doctor-patient relationship with someone they can see face to face and know and trust when required.

Does a Virtual Out-Patients Service Save Money?

The majority of out-patient encounters are financed not from one large pot of money that the Hospital or the health service shares, but through a series of transactions from the commissioners or health insurers per patient and per treatment or interaction type. Traditionally the Hospital then uses this money to pay its staff and its building maintenance costs and its overheads etc. Running a Hospital is an expensive business. Your average medium size Hospital spends about £3 million pounds per year on electricity for example.

A virtual hospital, however, does not have the same issues. There are minimal overheads. What you're paying for is the Consultant's expert specialist opinion and decision making, and that exists in their head and doesn't require the same infrastructure to provide. A virtual Hospital can deliver the same value to the system, for significantly less cost, say 60% of the standard tariff value or billing code, for the majority of the patients referred. This reflects an excellent cost saving for purchasers, tax payers and health services overall.

Does this mean that the Hospital then misses out? In one way that's correct, direct income from costly out-patient appointments may go down, with an associated reduction in footfall to the physical clinic. This then provides a smart opportunity for the Hospital to realise financial savings in other ways by reimagining their service around what really needs to take place there. Hospital services can coordinate the reallocation of capacity (in line with prominent health service initiatives) through a degree of transformation. No more expensive locum spending. No more out-sourcing of costly tests (such as endoscopies) or elective surgery to an external provider because they don't have enough in-house clinicians. Work can be repatriated, and this allows a lower cost way of delivering the same volume of essential activity that needs to take place in a physical setting. Overall income could go down but this does reflect savings for the wider health economy.

Ultimately virtual out-patient services save health services and payors money as they are cheaper to deliver and they reduce strain on the existing Hospital services, allowing them to focus on the more complex cases that need physical review and reduce their own internal cost pressures—so long as they are willing to undertake the service redesign work that stems from a new model of care. It's also a useful way of thinking about limiting cost growth in the medium to long term, because you take away the cost pressure of the demand on beleaguered services. If you think forwards, with costs going up every year, from a systems point of view, you minimise the growth and spend on out-patient services over time by being more sustainable and efficient. We can also get greater insights into understanding what degree of out-patient clinical activity we actually need to deliver physically, which is invaluable. The principle of the virtual model is to reduce the unnecessary demand on physical out-patient appointments such that the waiting times for the residual essential face to face services, are timelier and more accessible for those that need to attend.

What Do Patients Want?

In this data driven age when we are used to running our lives via the internet, banking, shopping, meetings, entertainment, it makes sense that many people would also want to manage their health issues in a convenient and accessible manner. Making an online booking for a medical appointment is much less hassle and time consuming for example, than actually having to phone the Doctors office. Self-service and access to our own medical information supports patient empowerment.

For virtual clinics to work effectively they need to be convenient and easy to use, allowing people to get the medical care from the comfort of their homes, or being minimally disruptive to their working lives. Quick and efficient healthcare with easy access to the right healthcare professional without having to travel or wait a long time provides a great deal of benefit and represents the type of patient expectation that health services should support in this era of digital health evolution. Coupled to this is the need for the same (or better) quality care that one might expect in a traditional out-patient service. Despite their convenience virtual health care services will quickly survive or fail based on how well they treat patients. Virtual offerings do have the advantage that they can provide access to a wider range of specialities and expert clinicians that might otherwise be available locally, especially if you are based outside of a major town or city. Quality also relates to the standard of communication being received, there is a push in the present for clinical correspondence to cut down on medical jargon and be directly addressed to the patient rather than their primary care Doctor, as they are the one who needs to understand what is going on with their care. Patients value clear and effective communication, their questions answered, and concerns addressed. It would also be good to receive any correspondence directly by email, rather than having to wait to be copied into a paper letter trail and get this several weeks down the line.

On the flip side, using virtual services for healthcare, there needs to be strong assurance and regulation around data privacy, information sharing and compliance. Most people are happy to review their financial information online but the outcomes of having our most personal medical data leaked via the internet could be devastating. In order to overcome future inequities in healthcare provision, there needs to be consideration around potentially digitally excluded populations of people, this could relate to everything from the user-friendliness of digital platforms, to not being able to access them at all because of lack of broadband availability or smart devices. Services such as Medefer however manage to obviate this by not placing any additional digital burden on the patient.

Two additional concerns relate to the nature of the medical interaction itself, given that it is care at one remove from the physical world, the lack of a hands on approach may cause some potential problems, firstly in terms of the relationship (there may not be one at all depending on how your problems are dealt with—being sent for a test and then discharged when the results come back negative), you may not feel able or willing to open up and explain what is really concerning you, or to put your full trust in the clinician and follow their recommendations, and this in turn can be harmful to your physical and mental wellbeing. And secondly, there is a worry that something could be missed. Reading a summary of a patients file or having a short phone or video call is not the same as being in the same room as them and this could limit the clinician's ability and thoroughness when it comes to their assessment. Careful and considered research is required to critically analyse the differences in outcomes, experience and satisfaction with the traditional model of care to make sure that we are not missing anything or making things worse for the sake of expediency.

Sample patient complaints and compliments about virtual medical services are shown below in Table 4.1.

The Future of Virtual Clinics

Use of technology to facilitate the work of out-patient clinics is likely to continue to grow given that both patients and providers can see the practical benefits and savings in costs. This will likely proceed down two main routes. The expansion of the use of telemedicine to replicate the traditional clinic encounter. Wider adoption means that this will become more mainstream and accepted as people become increasingly comfortable with telemedicine. Advances in technology will mean that systems can be more effective and when combined with remote monitoring tools there will be benefits relating to information gathering and accuracy. We may even

Table 4.1 Representative patient feedback relating to their experience of virtual out-patient services

Compliments	Complaints
Amazed at the speed at which my case was reviewed.	Nobody explained that I wouldn't get to see the Doctor
Had never been copied into my own clinical letters before so I finally got to understand what they were saying about me.	I was reviewed and discharged too quickly
So much better than having to go into the awful Hospital	Incredibly poor service on the support line
Very efficient, the service was really good. I would not hesitate to recommend to my family and friends. I am happy with the service I received.	I didn't know my referral would be sent to a third party.
Very positive experience for a test that isn't nice to think about. Very efficient, professional and excellent health care. I felt very reassured and was treated extremely well.	The letters were good but gave way too much information. I just wanted for the specialist to get on and deal with things.

see the development of VR headsets and cameras in order to provide a more immersive experience and enhance the elements of communication and interaction that may be lacking from some virtual clinic set ups.

The second route is that of using digital solutions to redesign the entire pathway of care from start to finish, for example breaking down the need for a primary care referral and allowing patients to access specialist care through self-service or criteria driven means (such as a bowel cancer identification programme). Disaggregating the need for a clinician to personally interact with every patient at every step of the journey allows them to use their time more efficiently. Using clinical AI to review test results as soon as they are completed will alert clinicians to concerning patterns of results. Integration with wearable tech and self-monitoring apps will support proactive and preventative care. Centralising specialist referrals so that they can be dealt with on a regional or even national level would allow scaling of such virtual approaches, a more even balancing of clinical capacity and demand, a reduction in care variation (obviating areas of poor practice) or even developing a global reach to support resource poor areas of the world.

Overall, the future of out-patient services will be shaped by patient experience and feedback, the need to control costs, along with changes in health policy, regulatory controls, technological sophistication and greater imagination about how we use the vital resource of Doctor's time and brains more efficiently.

References

1. Clark GN. A history of the royal college of physicians of London, vol. 2. London: Oxford University Press; 1966. p. 431.
2. Bridges R. St Bartholomew's Hospital reports, vol. 14. 1878. p. 167.

3. LCP Waiting list tracker. https://waitinglist.health.lcp.com/
4. World Population Review. Health care wait times by country 2024. https://worldpopulationreview.com/country-rankings/health-care-wait-times-by-country
5. Australian Medical Association. Shining a light on the elective surgery 'hidden' waiting list. https://www.ama.com.au/sites/default/files/2022-09/Shining%20a%20light%20on%20the%20elective%20surgery%20%27hidden%27%20waiting%20list.pdf
6. Engage Britain. Health and care survey. 2021 Sept. https://engagebritain.org/health-care-survey-experiences-nhs/
7. Medefer key outcomes. https://medefer.com/
8. Williamson T. Frimley ICB case study. https://xylaservices.com/about-xyla/case-studies/frimley-icb-case-study/
9. Open Medical case studies. https://www.openmedical.co.uk/case-studies
10. Greenhalgh T, Vijayaraghavan S, Wherton J, et al. Virtual online consultations: advantages and limitations (VOCAL) study. BMJ Open. 2016;6(1):e009388. https://doi.org/10.1136/bmjopen-2015-009388.

Further Reading

Loudon IS. Historical importance of out-patients. BMJ. 1978;1:974–7. https://www.bmj.com/content/bmj/1/6118/974.full.pdf

Chapter 5
The Rise of Virtual Primary Care

Abstract It is well recognised that primary care services are in high demand but are failing to provide enough capacity. Evolution of the primary care model holds immense promise. Virtual primary care could reshape the way healthcare is delivered, offering convenience, accessibility, and potential cost savings. As technology advances, the integration of artificial intelligence, machine learning, and predictive analytics will enhance diagnostic accuracy and more personalised treatment plans. Collaborations between virtual primary care providers and traditional healthcare institutions could create a hybrid model, combining the best of both worlds for patient care. While challenges exist, ongoing technological innovation and a patient-centred approach will likely drive the further expansion of virtual primary care, ultimately contributing to improved healthcare outcomes for individuals.

Keywords Primary care · General practice · General practitioners · Telemedicine · Triage and referral · Community care · Population health

A Cautionary Tale

Babylon the future of the NHS, goes into administration
Just announced!

Babylon Health, once the 'future of the NHS', goes into administration.

The UK AI health company touted by Matt Hancock was delisted by the New York Stock Exchange last month and has now called in the administrators

Babylon Health, the UK AI firm promoted as the future of the NHS by former health secretary Matt Hancock, has entered UK administration just 2 years after a high-profile listing on the New York Stock Exchange.

Babylon Health was delisted from the NYSE last month and is now facing collapse, after losing nearly all of its $4.2 billion valuation. The company's demise comes amid allegations of overhyped technology, questionable ties to the Conservative Party, and terminated contracts with UK hospitals.

Founded in 2013 by former UK Iranian banker Ali Parsa, Babylon claimed its AI could revolutionise healthcare through virtual appointments and diagnostic chatbots such as its GP at Hand, which it claims has 100,000 users in the UK. However, experts repeatedly warned the technology was unproven and overhyped.

Nevertheless, Babylon, which is registered in Jersey, won a number of NHS contracts, thanks in part to Hancock's promotion of GP at Hand in 2018.

Later, it was revealed that Babylon shareholders had donated £200,000 to the Conservative Party and Hancock's own leadership campaign in 2017 and 2018.

Hancock had said he wanted to see Babylon's digital first primary care service rolled out across the country. However, last August two NHS Trusts that had pioneered the system, Royal Wolverhampton NHS Trust and University Hospitals Birmingham NHS Foundation Trust said they were ending their multi-year contract with Babylon just 2 years after signing the deal.

Hammersmith and Fulham NHS Trust reportedly continues to operate the system.

Babylon went public in New York in 2021 at a $4.2 billion valuation, making Parsa a billionaire. But following the loss of Wolverhampton and Birmingham trusts, the company's share price fell by 85%.

In July 2023, in the face of continuing financial problems, Babylon was delisted from the NYSE. This month it announced that London-based investment firm AlbaCore Capital would take over its assets without shareholders' approval, and that it was calling in administrators in the UK.

In a statement on its website published 7th August, the company said it was in discussions to seek additional funding.

"Following Babylon's receipt of funding under its amended bridge notes facility with AlbaCore, Babylon has no binding commitment for additional financing to continue its business operations," the statement said.

"As a result, the Group is exploring new strategic alternatives in order to find the best possible outcome for its UK business," it continued.

"Babylon remains focused on continuing the day-to-day operations of its UK business, providing accessibility of its healthcare services and the highest standards of care for its patients and members. The Group is pursuing the divestiture of its UK business to third parties that may provide financing to assure the continuity of the operations."

The potential for AI to speed diagnostics and identify disease has long been touted as a primary use case for the technology, but while it is doubtless improving and can outperform human specialists in some areas, results have been patchy, occasionally producing false positives, false negatives and unpredictable outcomes.

> With the current levels of AI hype, Babylon's rapid fall from grace serves as a cautionary tale about the risks of overpromising untested healthcare technology, and of murky political lobbying.
>
> Two years after the blockbuster IPO that made its founder a billionaire, Babylon Health now faces bankruptcy and lawsuits from aggrieved investors.
>
> In an email to *Computing* a Babylon Health spokesperson said: "We want to emphasise that there will be no impact to the services we provide to our NHS GP at Hand, Direct-to-Consumer or Private patients and members. We will continue to uphold the highest standards of care and service for our patients and members."
>
> Box 5.1 Babylon News Story. Source: Computing World, August 2023 [1]. Reproduced with Permission.

This interesting summary of the fall of Babylon, illustrates the problems of the digital health buisnesses across the world (Box 5.1). An important component of the health ecosystem may have some transformative changes brought in, but if the technology doesn't work and fails to deliver on its promises and commercial greed gets in the way (like with Theranos), then it's destined to fail and there can be reactionary recoil for future investment and innovation, as well as detriments to patient care.

The Importance of Primary Care

Primary care is a fundamental and integral component of healthcare systems. It provides essential community-based healthcare services and focuses on promoting health, preventing disease, and managing common health issues and chronic conditions. For the majority of people, it provides the first point of contact with health services, acting as the 'front door' for the entire health system.

Primary Care Providers Include family physicians, general practitioners, community paediatricians, nurse practitioners, paramedics, and physician assistants. They are often the central point of contact for patients and oversee their overall healthcare on an ongoing basis ('cradle to grave').

Community Health Workers In many settings, community health workers, for example district nurses and health visitors play a vital role in connecting individuals with primary care services, especially in underserved communities.

Services Provided:
- Diagnosis and treatment of common illnesses and injuries.
- Routine check-ups and physical examinations.

- Management of chronic conditions (e.g., diabetes, hypertension).
- Health promotion and disease prevention (e.g., vaccinations, lifestyle counselling).
- Referrals to specialists when necessary.
- Coordination of care among different healthcare providers.
- Patient education and counselling on health-related matters.

Research has shown that access to primary health services and more widespread provision is linked to better overall health outcomes in a population, including improvements in self-rated health and a reduction in all-cause mortality [2]. As the main port of entry into the healthcare system, primary care providers are available to help individuals to understand and discuss their health and any particular problems that they may be experiencing. In case of more complex needs, as discussed in previous chapters, a referral can be made for more specialised care.

Characteristics of Primary Care

Primary care places a greater emphasis on the health of the whole person rather than a specific organ or system. This holistic approach contributes to positive effects such as reduced mortality rates due to the accumulated contribution of care, rather than the narrow focus of the specialist.

The close and ongoing relationship between patients and their primary care providers helps health professionals to understand their situation more completely and make relevant recommendations.

- **First Point of Contact:** Primary care is often the first place individuals go when they have health concerns or need medical advice.
- **Comprehensive Care:** Primary care covers a wide range of health needs, including general medical care, preventive services, health education, and management of chronic conditions.
- **Longitudinal Relationship:** Primary care providers often establish long-term relationships with their patients, which enables them to provide personalised and ongoing care. Primary care providers often develop long-term relationships with their patients, this fosters trust and enables the provider to have a comprehensive understanding of the patient's health history and needs.
- **Coordination:** Primary care providers coordinate a patient's care across various healthcare specialties and services, ensuring that all aspects of their health are managed in an organised manner.
- **Preventive Focus:** interventions such as vaccinations, screenings, and health education, are a core component of primary care, aimed at detecting problems early and keeping individuals healthy.

Primary care places a strong emphasis on preventive interventions that have an impact on many aspects of health, such as breastfeeding, stopping smoking, staying physically active and eating a healthy diet. In the United States, regions with a higher ratio of primary care physicians to population are positively correlated with reduced rates of smoking and obesity [3]. Additionally, it's been found that patients admitted to Hospital with complications related to a manageable health condition, such as hypertension, were four times more likely to lack access to a primary health care provider. When primary health practitioners are able to encourage preventative measures or make early interventions, referral to a specialist for disease-specific care can often be avoided, thus reducing the risks associated with treatment and reducing the burden on secondary care.

> *Primary healthcare is a whole-of-society approach to health that aims at ensuring the highest possible level of health and well-being and their equitable distribution by focusing on people's needs....as close as feasible to people's everyday environment.*—WHO and UNICEF [4]

In a joint report from the World Health Organisation and UNICEF, (A vision for primary health care in the twenty-first century: Towards Universal Health Coverage—UHC and the Sustainable Development Goals—SDGs) published in 2019 [4], some key statistics emerge relevant to primary care;

- About 930 million people worldwide are at risk of falling into poverty due to out-of-pocket health spending of 10% or more of their household budget.
- Scaling up primary health care (PHC) interventions across low and middle-income countries could save 60 million lives and increase average life expectancy by 3.7 years by 2030.
- Achieving the targets for PHC requires an additional investment of around US$ 200 to US$ 370 billion a year for a more comprehensive package of health services.
- At the UN high level UHC meeting in 2019, countries committed to strengthening primary health care. The WHO recommends that every country allocate or reallocate an additional 1% of GDP to PHC from government and external funding sources.

It can be argued that for health coverage to be truly universal, a shift is needed from health systems designed around diseases and institutions towards health systems designed for people, by people. Primary care requires Governments at all levels to reinforce the importance of action beyond the health sector in order to pursue a whole-of government approach to health, including health-in-all-policies, a strong focus on equity and interventions that encompass the entire life-course.

Challenges in Primary Care

Primary care unfortunately faces several significant issues, many of which can impact the quality, accessibility, and effectiveness of healthcare delivery. Some of the main issues facing primary care include:

Shortage of Primary Care Providers Many regions, particularly rural and underserved areas, experience a shortage of primary care physicians, nurse practitioners, and physician assistants. This shortage can lead to limited access to care and longer wait times for appointments. Not enough Doctors are being trained and general practice is seen as a less attractive speciality given the long hours and heavy workload. There are disincentives for trained clinicians to go and work in particular areas, especially if there are few other practitioners locally and the burden of responsibility will fall on them, meaning that they have to be available more frequently to cover out of hours shifts and weekends. It's not unusual to see advertisements for highly remunerated GP posts in remote places such as Canada or New Zealand, or on far away islands, which want to attract Doctors to work in the wilderness.

The Ageing Population We're all living longer thanks to better sanitation, vaccinations, health and safety practices and modern medicine. But this means that the burden of disease grows as we stay alive longer and accumulate more illnesses along the way. As populations age, the demand for primary care services increases due to the prevalence of chronic conditions and complex healthcare needs. A 2017 study by Mini and Thankappan from the Centre for Public health at the Amrita Institute of Medical Sciences in India, showed that overall, 63% of older adults suffered from at-least one non-communicable disease and 30.7% of them had multimorbidity [5]. The most common combination of morbidities were, high blood pressure and arthritis (7.5%), cataracts and arthritis (5.3%) and high blood pressure and diabetes (4.7%). Meeting the healthcare demands of an ageing population can significantly strain the resources of primary care.

Workforce Burnout Primary care providers often experience high levels of burnout due to heavy workloads, administrative burdens, and the emotional toll of caring for patients with chronic illnesses. Burnout can lead to decreased job satisfaction and provider shortages. In a study of the prevalence of GP burnout rates across the world by Christo Karuna of Monash Business School published in 2022, it was found that internationally there were much higher than average rates of emotional exhaustion, depersonalisation and low personal accomplishment, all contributing to high levels of stress and burnout [6]. Primary Care Doctors often highlight the unpaid invisible workload of the inbox, emails and paperwork, relating to both patient care and running a business, undertaken in their own time in the evenings and over weekends and holidays. This causes a negative spiral of exhaustion and anxiety, a fear of missing a significant result or diagnosis and eventually, severe effects on mental health.

Healthcare Disparities Disparities in access to care and health outcomes persist, with vulnerable populations, such as low-income individuals and racial or ethnic minorities, often facing barriers to accessing decent primary care services. Additional contributors are the decisions made by the local care boards and health authorities that make spending decisions about what kind of healthcare provision takes place in a region, this is often referred to as the postcode lottery. Addressing these disparities is a significant challenge.

Healthcare Costs The rising cost of healthcare, including insurance premiums, co-payments, and deductibles, can deter individuals from seeking care, leading to delayed or deferred input. Several countries around the world make a charge for accessing primary care and this acts as a barrier of entry to many.

Fragmented Care Lack of care coordination and communication among different healthcare providers can lead to fragmented care, which may result in delays, medical errors, duplicated tests, and suboptimal patient outcomes. This is exacerbated by lack of technical integration of IT systems and issues with interoperability. Medical data is held in siloes and this leads to confusion, delays, communication failures and problems with instigating treatments as arguments persist over who is responsible and who pays for what.

Regulatory and Payment Reforms Frequent changes in healthcare regulations and payment models can create uncertainty for primary care practices. Shifting reimbursement structures and contracts may affect the financial viability of primary care providers. There is a big move away from the GP partnership model in the UK as it is becoming less economically viable for practitioners.

Patient Engagement Encouraging patients to actively participate in their healthcare, adhere to treatment plans, and adopt healthier lifestyles can be challenging. Low health literacy and the social determinants of health can influence patient engagement.

Mental Health Integration Integrating mental health services into primary care settings is essential, as mental health issues are common within the general population. However, this integration requires additional resources and training for general practitioners and their teams.

Preventive Care and Health Education Promoting preventive care and health education to prevent chronic diseases and promote overall wellness can be challenging, especially when competing with the demands of acute care.

Technological Challenges While technology can enhance primary care, the adoption of electronic health records (EHRs) and other health information technologies can be challenging and time-consuming for providers. Interoperability issues can hinder the exchange of patient data between healthcare systems. For example, while telemedicine offers benefits, its successful implementation requires addressing issues related to technology accessibility, licensing, reimbursement, and ensuring equitable access for all patients.

Tackling the above challenges requires a multi-faceted approach, including healthcare policy reforms, increased investment in primary care, expanded training and workforce development, improved care coordination, efforts to reduce healthcare disparities and digital solutions. As primary care serves as the foundation of healthcare systems, addressing these challenges is crucial for improving the overall health and well-being of populations (Fig. 5.1).

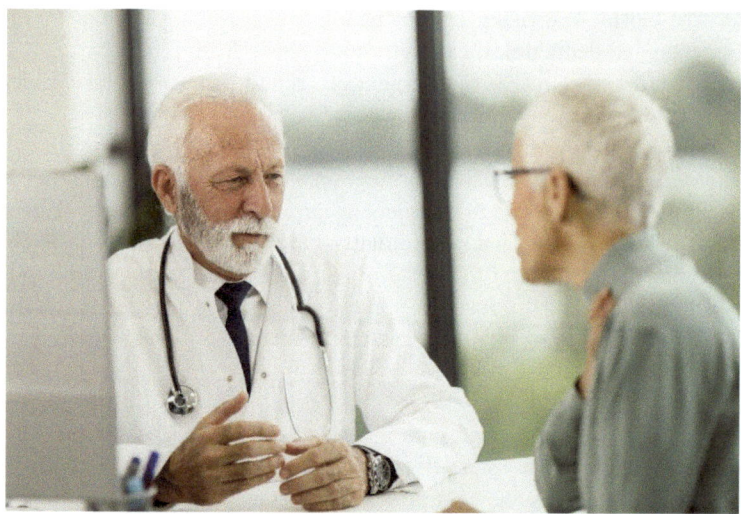

Fig. 5.1 Face to face patient consultation. Credit: Direct Media. Reproduced under StockSnap's Creative Commons CC0 Licence. https://creativecommons.org/publicdomain/zero/1.0/ (unmodified from Source: https://stocksnap.io/photo/doctor-patient-N9YCBA2UBU)

The Evolution of Primary Care

These challenges and pressures to change have had an impact, including recognition of the greater need for technology. With the advent of digital health solutions such as electronic messaging and telemedicine, patients can now consult with primary care providers remotely, breaking down geographic barriers, improving convenience, and expanding healthcare access. This section delves into the world of virtual primary care, exploring its evolution, benefits, potential downsides, and the future it holds for healthcare delivery.

'Virtual primary care' refers to the delivery of primary healthcare services remotely, through digital platforms and communication tools. It encompasses a range of services typically provided by a Primary Care Doctor, including medical consultations, diagnoses, prescriptions, preventive care, and follow-up visits. Making use of video calls, chatbots on their websites or via an App, wearable devices, and data analytics, virtual primary care offers patients access to medical expertise from the comfort of their homes, and hopefully relieves some of the pressures outlined above.

This evolution has occurred in light of a variety of factors;

Electronic Health Records (EHRs) EHRs have transformed primary care by digitising patient records, making them more easily accessible to healthcare providers. This enables better coordination of care, reduces errors, and improves patient outcomes. However, such systems do not always effectively integrate with secondary care or other locally based services, and this is a major barrier that needs to be overcome to avoid medical data being locked away in siloes. What is required is greater interoperability standards between systems.

Telemedicine Development Telemedicine has been in use for decades, primarily in remote areas or for specialist consultations. The increased acceptability of tele-communication technologies facilitates the exchange of medical information between patients and healthcare providers and makes it easier and more convenient to see their family Doctor—or an alternative provider such as Babylon (as was).

Digital Transformation The widespread adoption of electronic health records, mobile devices, and high-speed internet additionally paved the way for the integration of other technologies and new ways of working such as electronic prescribing into primary care practices. Healthcare providers began offering virtual visits as a convenient alternative to in-person consultations and the trend is likely to continue.

Expansion of Services Virtual primary care services have expanded to include a wide range of healthcare needs, such as routine check-ups, chronic disease management, mental health counselling, and preventive care. The COVID-19 pandemic accelerated the adoption of virtual care as safety concerns limited in-person visits.

As technology continues to advance, the future of digitally enabled virtual primary care looks promising. Key developments already being used include:

Remote Monitoring The integration of wearable devices and IoT (Internet of Things) technology will enable continuous remote monitoring of patients' vital signs and health metrics. For example home blood pressure monitoring kits enable regular home testing (avoiding the need for patients to come in to the practice) and data can be shared and analysed electronically which allows the identification of trends over time in order to pick up worrying changes that would have previously required intervention and potential hospitalisation.

Mobile Health (mHealth) Apps Mobile apps offer patients tools to monitor their health, track medications, and receive personalised health information. They can also help healthcare providers communicate with patients more effectively. A good example of this form of digital therapeutics is 'MySugr' which is used for the management of type 1 and type 2 diabetes (Fig. 5.2 below). It offers carbohydrate counting, glucose tracking and facilitates medication (insulin) dose calculation, it is able to generate longitudinal reports on glucose levels and allows sharing of data with the Doctor.

Population Health Management Tools The use of data analytics and risk identification tools help primary care providers uncover at-risk populations so that they can proactively get in touch and develop preventive strategies designed to improve overall community health.

Fig. 5.2 Snapshot of the
MySugr digital
therapeutics App. . Source:
MySugr.com © 2023
mySugr GmbH

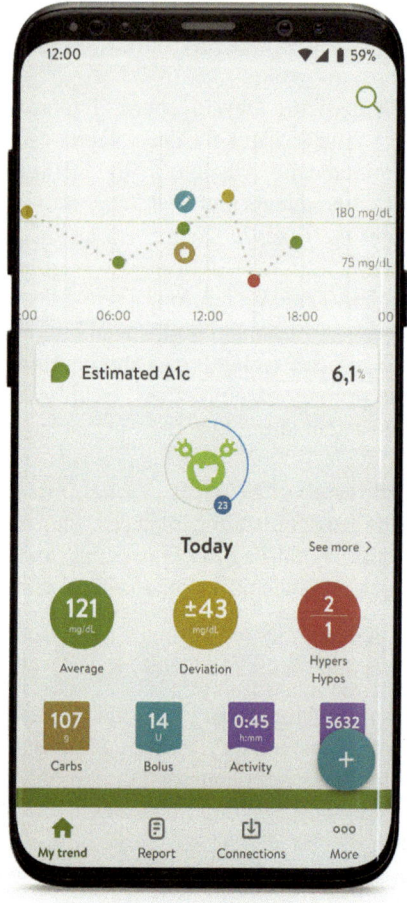

Patient Portals Primary care is increasingly providing a secure platform (such as
Patient Knows Best) for patients to access their own medical records, schedule
appointments, and communicate with healthcare providers (eConsult). Online
booking systems and automated appointment reminders improve patient attendance
and reduce no-show rates. Access to information promotes greater engagement and
understanding from the patient perspective. Linked to this are opportunities to navigate patients to online education and self-management resources.

Electronic Prescribing E-prescribing systems enable healthcare providers to send
prescriptions directly to pharmacies (or even the patient's home), reducing
medication errors, streamlining the prescription process and overcoming paperwork
based delays (Fig. 5.3).

These technologies have played a crucial role in improving primary care by
increasing accessibility, enhancing communication, and supporting evidence-based

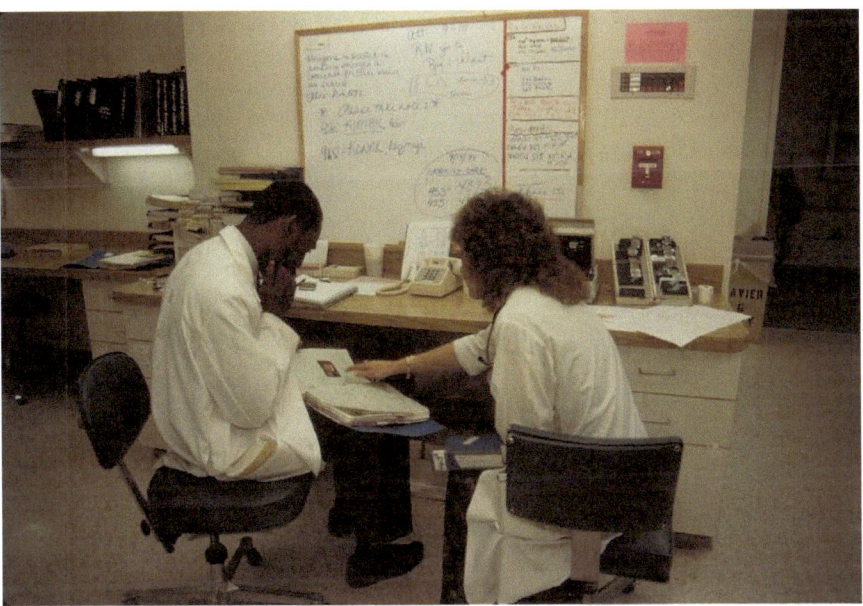

Fig. 5.3 Many Doctors around the world are still heavily paper based, especially when it comes to prescriptions. Credit: Martha Cooper. Source: Picryl.com (https://picryl.com/media/doctors-and-nurses-at-the-oncology-nurses-station-4th-floor-4). Reproduced under GetArchive Content Licence Agreement

decision-making in healthcare systems around the world. Such systems play an important role in helping Doctors manage more patients remotely, stay on top of their workload and all of the many tasks that they are responsible for. But there's even more exciting developments on the horizon.

Decision Support Tools Clinical decision support systems are a software or information system designed to assist healthcare providers, including doctors, nurses, and other clinicians, in making clinical decisions and providing patient care. These tools are typically based on a combination of medical knowledge, patient data, and best practices and guidelines, and they are used to improve the quality, safety, and efficiency of healthcare delivery. Clinical decision support tools can take various forms, including standalone software applications, integrated modules within EHR systems, or mobile apps. They can assist healthcare providers in making evidence-based decisions by providing access to the latest medical research and guidelines.

Artificial Intelligence (AI) and Machine Learning AI-driven tools can analyse vast amounts of healthcare data to identify patterns, drug interactions, predict disease outbreaks, and assist with more accurate and efficient diagnosis and treatment planning. The analysis of large datasets can provide insights into population health trends, improve decision-making, and help in the identification of high-risk patient groups.

Health Information Exchange (HIE) Better systems integration will facilitate the secure sharing of patient data between different healthcare providers (as well as the patient and their carers), this will enable improved care coordination, digital transfers of care and reduce confusion, duplications and delays. Enhanced interoperability between healthcare systems will ensure seamless sharing of patient data across different providers and platforms. Such standards are something that need to be mandated by system overlords.

Advanced Primary Care IT systems Currently most primary care IT applications are clunky databases that are hard to navigate and don't speak to other systems. Newer systems such as EMIS-X for example do more for the primary care Doctor by actively listening in, recording and interpreting the medical consultation. By picking out key words through speech recognition such as 'chest pain' the system can automatically bring up the latest treatment guidelines and summarise the meeting without the Doctor having to spend so much time inputting data into the computer and getting distracted during patient interactions.

Benefits of the Virtual Primary Care Approach

The adoption of virtual primary care has brought about numerous benefits to practitioners, patients, healthcare providers, and the healthcare system as a whole, and it is hoped that the addition of further digital health solutions will continue this trend. Virtual primary care, which involves undertaking more remote work has the advantage of eliminating geographical barriers, meaning that people in isolated or underserved areas, or those with limited mobility, that did not have access to a family Doctor, can now receive healthcare which was not previously possible for them. Virtual methods thus address healthcare disparities in rural and remote areas where access to in-person care can be limited. Patients in these regions can receive timely healthcare services without having to travel long distances. Added to this is the convenience of being able to book and schedule appointments at more flexible times and this avoids the rush of trying to get through on the telephone first thing in the morning along with everyone else, reducing the need for travel and time off work or school, as well as time and cost savings. This convenience can lead to better patient compliance with appointments and care plans because there is lesser overall frustration with the system. Virtual primary care allows patients to consult with their Doctor from the privacy and comfort of their homes. This can be particularly valuable for individuals with sensitive or stigmatised health concerns.

One important aspect of virtual care is that it helps to maintain continuity of care by enabling a consistent relationship between patient and their Doctor, even when physical visits aren't possible. This continuity of care can lead to better health outcomes and a deeper understanding of individual patient needs. Virtual primary care is well-suited for managing chronic conditions. Patients with conditions like diabetes, hypertension, or asthma can receive ongoing monitoring, medication management, and lifestyle counselling through virtual visits, navigation to self-management and education resources, and the benefits of information sharing through a patient portal or shared care record mean that patients are more likely to be engaged and activated with regards to their health over time. There is a great deal of evidence to show that patient education and health promotion through telehealth platforms, empowers patients to make informed decisions about their health. Use of technology can lead to enhanced communication. Technology, such as secure messaging and telehealth platforms, can improve communication between patients and providers. Patients may find it more convenient to reach out to their healthcare team for questions or concerns.

Finally, there are the potential benefits from greater integration of tech. Virtual primary care can incorporate remote monitoring devices, enabling healthcare providers to track patients' vital signs and progress, particularly for those with chronic conditions. Remote monitoring and data analysis enable healthcare providers to identify health trends and intervene early, preventing the progression of certain conditions. Such an approach allows earlier detection of negative changes which supports proactive care and the avoidance of Hospital admissions.

Challenges and Considerations

Whilst virtual and remote primary care holds significant promise, it also faces several challenges. Not all primary care facilities and certainly not all patients have access to the necessary technology, digital devices or internet connectivity for virtual care, potentially exacerbating healthcare disparities. There are obvious clinical limitations, some aspects of physical examinations and diagnostic tests cannot be replicated in virtual care settings, necessitating in-person visits. Additionally, the quality of clinical assessment may be very variable. Certain medical conditions and symptoms require a physical examination to make an accurate diagnosis. Virtual visits may limit healthcare providers' ability to observe non-verbal cues and physical manifestations of illness, potentially affecting diagnostic accuracy. The lack of examination when consulting remotely could lead to potential misdiagnoses or oversights and this could lead to a low threshold for organising an additional face-to-face consultation or specialist referral as a safety net. Patients with complex medical conditions or multiple comorbidities may require more in-depth assessments and coordination of care, which can be challenging to achieve through virtual care alone. Up to a third of GP appointments are now conducted virtually—primarily over the phone—and researchers from the University of Oxford have suggested that serious incidents or harm caused by remote consultations were rare and that the vast majority were safe [7]. When errors do happen, they commonly tend to be related to a missed diagnosis or underestimating the severity of a condition. They did suggest that Doctors shouldn't give telephone or virtual appointments to patients who are elderly, deaf or technophobes, which makes sense.

Alongside this, the absence of physical interactions may negatively impact the Doctor-patient relationship (that cornerstone of therapeutics, the building of trust and rapport) and the empathetic aspect of care that so many patients, including the most vulnerable in our society, need and cherish, especially in the most sensitive and complex medical situations. Some patients may be less engaged or motivated in virtual care compared to in-person care, potentially leading to lower adherence to treatment plans or lifestyle modifications. From a practical perspective there is also the potential for an increased administrative burden from poorly designed digital systems. Electronic health records and administrative tasks associated with technology can consume a significant portion of a provider's time, leaving less time for direct patient care and building relationships, if they have a poor user experience or are dysfunctional.

Importantly, virtual primary care is not suitable for emergency medical situations that require immediate attention. Patients experiencing severe symptoms or emergencies must be directed to seek in-person care. It's important to recognise that virtual primary care is not a one-size-fits-all solution and is best suited for certain types of visits and medical conditions. Patients with limited technology literacy may struggle to engage effectively in virtual care, potentially leading to frustration and misunderstandings. Hybrid models of care that combine virtual and in-person visits can help address many of these limitations while still leveraging the benefits of virtual primary care for routine and follow-up appointments.

The Loss of the Caring Relationship?

Is the caring relationship in primary care being lost because of the use of more technology?

The use of technology in healthcare, including within primary care, can have both positive and negative effects on the relationship between patients and their Doctors. While technology offers numerous benefits, it can also create challenges in maintaining a strong and compassionate patient-provider relationship. Technology can impact the interaction with a family Doctor because an over-reliance on technology can reduce personal experience, making it hard for clinicians to develop a strong relationship with their patients. Virtual consultations can lack the personal touch and empathy that can be conveyed through physical presence. Miscommunications can occur through virtual means, and important non-verbal cues may be missed, potentially impacting the quality of the interaction. This can be exacerbated by patients with low levels of digital literacy who may struggle to engage effectively in virtual care, potentially leading to frustration and misunderstandings. Furthermore, the extensive use of technology, including automation, self-service and AI driven tools may inadvertently lead to dehumanisation and patients feeling like they are being treated as cogs in a process, rather than unique individuals with needs and emotions.

To maintain a strong caring relationship in primary care while utilising technology healthcare providers should be mindful of the following:

Balancing Technology with Personal Interaction Healthcare providers should aim to strike a balance between using technology for efficiency and maintaining personal, compassionate interactions during in-person visits. Ongoing feedback from patient representatives and user groups and analysis of clinical incidents and complaints data will help systems to respond iteratively.

Patient Education Health services need to educate patients about the benefits and limitations of technology in healthcare, addressing any concerns and building trust.

Training and Communication Skills Doctors may benefit from additional training in effective communication and empathy, especially in virtual care settings, to convey warmth and understanding through digital means, and address the emotional aspects of healthcare.

Empathetic Virtual Communication During virtual visits, providers should make an effort to convey empathy and actively listen to patients to ensure they feel heard and cared for. One of the benefits of new technology systems (for example CliniScriber—a system that takes clinical notes and using AI composes them into a standardised set of medical notes with a differential diagnosis and outline management plan) is that they will actually allow clinicians to spend more time in direct patient care and reduce the computer related administration and data collection that has become so common in modern medical interactions [8]. *"I feel like I cheated"* reported Consultant Endocrinologist Dr. Ken Laji, after using such a system, *"One doesn't have to make constant notes and hold a load of information in your head and then rush to get it down - the system does it for you. It means that I can just concentrate on having a conversation"* [9].

Ultimately, technology should be viewed as a tool that can enhance relationships when used thoughtfully. It is up to Doctors to adapt to these changes and find ways to maintain a strong caring relationship in the age of digital healthcare. Meanwhile policy makers and health service payors need to support primary care with the best funding and support of technology implementation to help overcome the many challenges that can get in the way of good patient care and improved outcomes.

Summary

Virtual primary care represents a transformative shift in healthcare delivery, offering improved access, convenience, and cost-efficiency. As the field continues to evolve and address its challenges, it has the potential to become a cornerstone of healthcare delivery, improving the overall health and well-being of individuals worldwide. Embracing virtual primary care is not just an option for the future but a necessity in ensuring healthcare access and quality for all. While virtual primary care offers many benefits, it's essential to address challenges such as technology access and privacy concerns to ensure equitable access and high-quality care for all patients. As technology continues to advance, virtual primary care has the potential to play an increasingly prominent role in modern healthcare systems.

References

1. Leonard J. Babylon Health, once the 'future of the NHS', goes into administration. Computing World. 2023. https://www.computing.co.uk/news/4121796/babylon-health-future-nhs-goes-administration#:~:text=Babylon%20Health%2C%20the%20UK%20AI,the%20New%20York%20S...
2. Starfield B, Shi L, Macinko J. Contribution of primary care to health systems and health. Milbank Q. 2005;83(3):457–502. https://doi.org/10.1111/j.1468-0009.2005.00409.x.
3. Nielsen M, Langner B, Zema C, Hacker T, Grundy P. Benefits of implementing the primary care patient centered medical home: a review of cost and quality results 2012. https://thepcc.org/sites/default/files/media/benefits_of_implementing_the_primary_care_pcmh.pdf
4. World Health Organisation and Unicef. A vision for primary health care in the 21st century: towards UHC and the SDGs. 2019. https://www.who.int/docs/default-source/primary-health/vision.pdf
5. Mini GK, Thankappan KR. Pattern, correlates and implications of non-communicable disease multimorbidity among older adults in selected Indian states: a cross-sectional study. BMJ Open. 2017;7:e013529. https://doi.org/10.1136/bmjopen-2016-013529.
6. Karuna C, Palmer V, Scott A, Gunn J. Prevalence of burnout among GPs: a systematic review and meta-analysis. Br J Gen Pract. 2022;72(718):e316–24. https://doi.org/10.3399/BJGP.2021.0441.
7. Payne R, Clarke A, Swann N, et al. Patient safety in remote primary care encounters: multi-method qualitative study combining Safety I and Safety II analysis. BMJ Qual Saf. Published Online First: 2023 Nov 28; https://doi.org/10.1136/bmjqs-2023-016674.
8. https://cliniscriber.com/
9. Personal communication.

Further Reading

Shi L. Primary care assessment tools. Johns Hopkins Bloomberg School of Public Health. Primary Care Policy Center. https://publichealth.jhu.edu/johns-hopkins-primary-care-policy-center/primary-care-assessment-tools
The fall of Babylon: failed telehealth startup once valued at $2B goes bankrupt, sold for parts. https://techcrunch.com/2023/08/31/the-fall-of-babylon-failed-tele-health-startup-once-valued-at-nearly-2b-goes-bankrupt-and-sold-for-parts/?guccounter=1

Chapter 6
The Virtual Emergency Department

Abstract In today's fast-paced world, the concept and reach of emergency care delivery is evolving rapidly. Traditional emergency rooms and urgent care centres are often crowded, busy and chaotic, leading to long wait times and delayed access to critical medical attention. To address these challenges, virtual emergency care, using new technologies, has emerged as a revolutionary solution. This chapter delves into the realm of virtual emergency care, exploring its development, benefits, challenges, and future prospects.

Keywords Accident and emergency · Emergency department · Triage and referral · Care navigation · Prioritisation · Waiting times · Remote consultations

Handling Emergencies

Accidents and emergencies are a staple ingredient of Hospital based care delivery. The emergency room (ER) or emergency department (ED) is a receiving point for all manner of acute illnesses and trauma, acting a triaging funnel to sort patients into the right care buckets and swiftly treat medical and surgical emergencies. However, its capacity to cope does not always meet demand, especially during the winter months when the perfect storm of viral respiratory illnesses and weather-related trauma, amongst other factors, precipitate a major squeeze on its ability to manage (Fig. 6.1).

According to the Centres for Disease Control, nearly 139 million patients attend emergency rooms in the USA each year [1]. The commonest types of medical problems that present themselves are injuries, poisoning, respiratory issues, circulatory conditions, digestive problems, musculo-skeletal disorders (aches and pains) and genito-urinary problems. Interestingly only 14% of patient visits resulted in Hospital admission (61 per 1000 population). The majority (86%) resulted in treatment and release, and in this category the main illnesses were upper respiratory tract infections, non-specific chest pains, abdominal pains, diarrhoea and digestive problems.

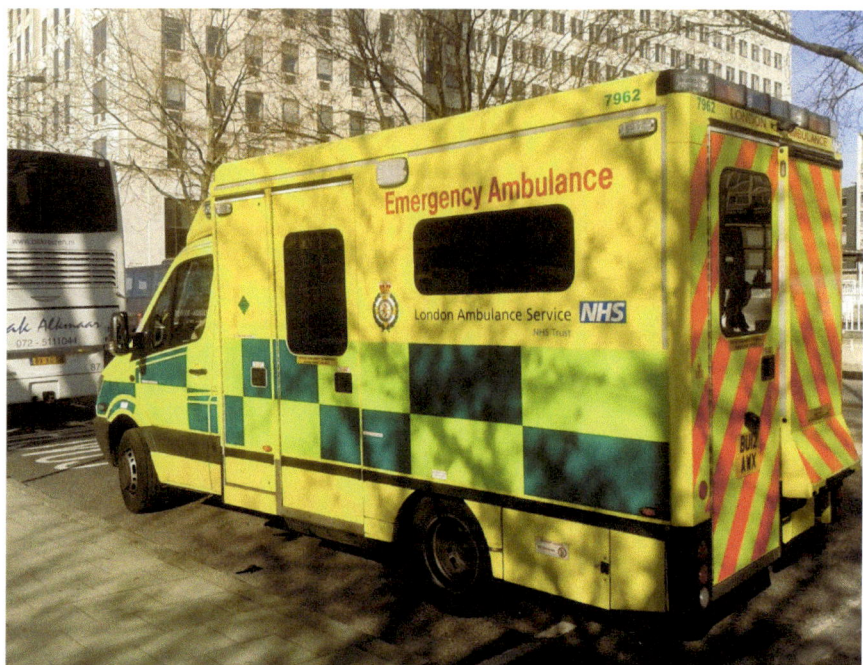

Fig. 6.1 Ambulance queues and delays, a common scene outside many emergency departments. Image Source: PxHere (https://pxhere.com/en/photo/493283) Reproduced under Creative Commmons Public Domain Licence 1.0 (https://creativecommons.org/publicdomain/zero/1.0/)

In the UK, there is a national target that 95% of ED patients should be seen, treated, discharged or admitted within a time frame of 4 hours. Performance against this target has dropped off significantly over recent years as the demands on A&E departments have grown (including people not being able to access primary care help) (see Fig. 6.2 below).

Back in 2019, a large public engagement exercise entitled 'The Big Conversation' was undertaken across Cambridgeshire in the UK, by the local urgent and emergency care collaborative to find out people's preferences for how emergency care should be designed and delivered [2]. This pre-pandemic survey revealed that;

- 79% of people wanted to access healthcare faster, through technology.
- 88% of people believed that individuals should be re-directed to other services, if they went to an ED and did not have serious injuries or illnesses.
- 73% wanted advice about treatment, and the ability to book an appointment within a short time span.

A significant portion of ED visits are for non-emergency or primary care issues. Treating non-urgent cases in the ED can strain resources and drive up healthcare costs. Overcrowding and resource constraints can lead to delayed care for those with critical conditions and there are low levels of overall patient satisfaction.

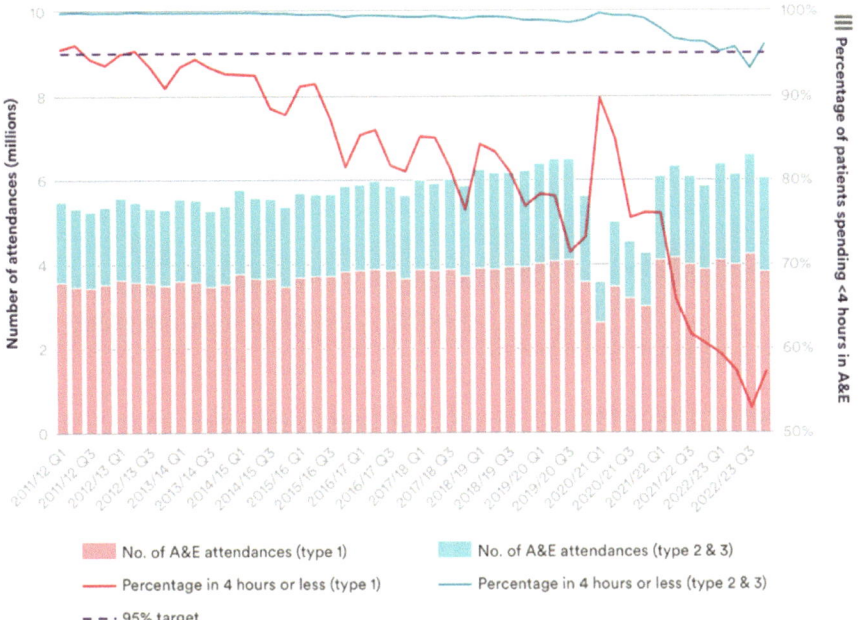

Fig. 6.2 QualityWatch analysis of NHS England A&E attendance data. Unmodified. Image Source: The Nuffield Trust (https://www.nuffieldtrust.org.uk/resource/a-e-waiting-times)

Additionally, patients with mental health crises frequently attend the ED, but they may lack the specialised staff and facilities needed to provide appropriate psychiatric care. This all takes it toll on the healthcare professionals. ED staff often face high levels of stress due to the fast-paced environment, critical cases, and frequent exposure to trauma which can lead to burnout and high levels of turnover.

> *There is a lack of appreciation outside emergency departments and the ambulance service about how difficult the current situation is and how this stifles innovation*—Consultant in Emergency Medicine [2]

How Can Emergency Care Be Delivered Differently?

If you consider 'out of hospital' cardiac arrests—a common enough occurrence that we are now familiar with the sight of defibrillators on the high street and an awareness of the concept of CPR (cardio-pulmonary resuscitation)—then it's fascinating to see how a combination of integrated technology can make a significant difference.

If you are unfortunate enough to suffer an unexpected cardiac arrest (essentially your heart stopping and no longer being alive) then your chances of survival (being successfully resuscitated and coming back to life) are approximately 9%. If this happens in a built-up environment, such as a modern airport, then your survival

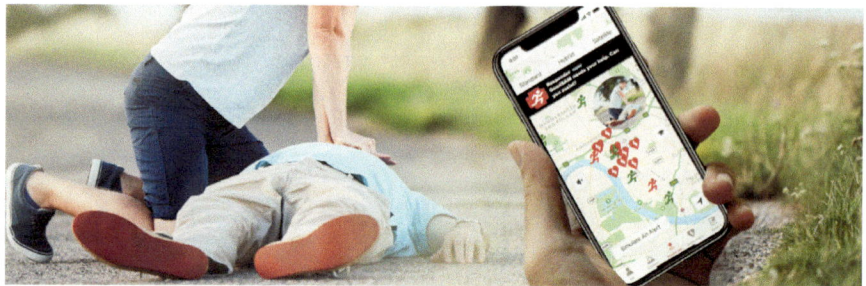

Fig. 6.3 Bystander CPR in action. Reproduced with permission from GoodSAM (https://www.goodsamapp.org/alertingAndDispatching)

rates goes up significantly to around 80%. This is because there are far more CPR trained staff and crew around and there are defibrillators at every other gate. The difference in survival is due to eliminating the time delay in starting emergency treatments such as CPR (Fig. 6.3).

The GoodSam platform seeks to connect specialist expertise with hyper locality [3]. It does this by alerting people who are nearby to an incident (such as a collapse or a head injury) to get there quickly and take immediate life saving measures such as maintaining the individual's airway or starting chest compressions, before the ambulance has even arrived. The principle is around combining community crowd-sourcing and technology to try and increase survival from cardiac arrest. It's a system that alerts people who are registered on the platform (such as off-duty Doctors, Nurses, Police Officers, Firemen, Paramedics—people who are trained in CPR) and they get notified by the ambulance services to incidents close by (through geolocation) and informed where abouts the person is that needs their emergency help. They can often make their way to the incident and be there much quicker (as they are already in the vicinity) than the ambulance. For every minute that you start doing CPR earlier, the chances of survival increase by 10%. Research has shown that being attended by a GoodSAM Responder increased the odds ratio for survival to hospital discharge by 3.19 in London and 3.15 in the East Midlands—a significant improvement [4].

The technology can also be used to help emergency dispatcher's triage incidents and provide immediate support remotely. When you call for an ambulance from your smartphone the emergency services may send you a text notification to request temporary sharing of your location data and access to your video camera. If you accept, then this can be shared with a healthcare professional on the other end of the line who'll then be able to see what you can see via your phone camera [5]. The system can analyse visual information from the patients face, using AI, to measure their pulse and respiratory rate, so that vital signs can be remotely picked up. The key research findings of an analysis of 838 emergency GoodSAM Instant-On-Scene Videos showed that;

- The use of GoodSAM video interaction changed the assessment of the patient's condition in 51.1% of calls—12.9% more critical, 38.2% less critical.
- GoodSAM video altered the emergency response in 27.5% of cases.
- Quality of care (e.g. CPR or airway control) improved in 28.4% of calls with GoodSAM Video.
- 97.3% of callers felt live video should be implemented.

A Virtual Emergency Department

There is a pressing need to work differently in order to take the strain off the ED and reduce avoidable attendance. The idea of providing medical advice and consultation remotely has gained traction as technologies have advanced. The emergence of high-speed internet, mobile devices, and the proliferation of video conferencing platforms and their increased adoption opens up new possibilities for healthcare providers to see patients at a remove and still provide good quality accessible and convenient care.

Telemedicine services were initially used for non-emergency consultations, but their potential for emergency care became evident during crises like natural disasters and pandemics, where traditional healthcare systems struggled to cope with the surge in patient demand. One of the major benefits is that clinicians from further afield can be pulled in to provide additional capacity that would not otherwise be readily accessible.

Research by NHS England [6] suggests that;

- >20% of patients presenting with minor injuries could be diverted to either an alternative, less acute setting (Urgent Treatment Centre (UTC)), primary care, their local pharmacy or to self-care, if they were able to be fully assessed via video consultation by a clinician with a special interest in the management of minor injuries, or
- >20% of patients could be diverted from the Emergency Department (ED) if they were similarly fully assessed by an experienced Emergency Department Consultant or Specialist Doctor.

This line of thinking pushes services in the direction of greater upfront and remote assessment. A virtual emergency department is therefore a healthcare service that provides emergency medical care remotely using telemedicine and digital technologies. It's designed to offer immediate assistance and evaluation to patients who may be experiencing urgent medical issues but do not require a physical presence in the traditional ED setting. The virtual ED model relieves the burden on emergency departments through a number of key approaches;

- Virtually managing and discharging appropriate patients, preventing ED in-person attendances.
- Directing patients needing urgent emergency care to the ED and, where possible, streamlining their ED journey, for example, direct admission to the surgical care unit.

- Redirecting patients needing less urgent specialist care to outpatient clinics bypassing the ED altogether eg. fracture clinics.
- Redistribute patient time of arrival by scheduling their ED care to less busy times.

Here's how a virtual emergency department typically functions:

Remote Consultations Patients can access the virtual emergency department through online platforms or dedicated apps. They complete screening questions to ensure that they are not imminently dying and then after being queued, connect with healthcare professionals, such as Doctors, Nurse Practitioners, or Paramedics, via video calls, audio calls, or online chat. These clinicians may be local or work in another part of the country entirely as part of a distributed network. During the virtual consultation, healthcare providers assess the patient's symptoms, medical history, and vital signs. They use this information to determine the level of urgency and the appropriate course of action.

Treatment Recommendations Based on the triage and assessment, the healthcare provider may offer medical advice, prescribe medications, recommend self-care measures, or suggest further diagnostic tests or consultations. They can also guide patients on when it is necessary to seek in-person care as a form of safety netting.

The use of a video consultations makes it possible for patients to have the first part of their care delivered at home. Often this can result in a different and more efficient journey. For example, a patient with suspected broken wrist can be sent straight for an X-ray before attending an urgent treatment centre rather than the normal ED and having to wait around. The mother of a young child who has swallowed a foreign body can be reassured that they don't need to come to the ED but can instead let nature take its course. Patients can also be directed to other suitable alternative locations such as minor injury units, pharmacies, GP's, dentists or even given advice and guidance or resources about self-care. For patients who do need a diagnostic test such as a scan, they can be directed to the radiology department to have this done before having to hang about in the ED, saving patients (and the system) time waiting and reducing congestion in the ED waiting rooms. They can also arrange for immediate referral to the right speciality e.g. Gynaecology or Surgery, completely bypassing the ED, where appropriate.

Emergency Response Coordination In situations where immediate in-person care is required, the virtual ED can help coordinate an ambulance or direct the patient to the nearest physical emergency room and notify the department to expect them so that they can bypass the normal queue. The virtual ED acts as a form of care navigation, getting the patient into the right part of the health system—which may not always be an ED. This can work very well if the managing clinicians or administrators have insights into how busy various ED's are in an area so can direct the patient accordingly and provide a level of seriousness rating (e.g. Red/Amber/Green) so it's clear how urgently they should be dealt with.

Follow-Up Care Virtual emergency departments can also often offer after care options, allowing patients to schedule virtual consultations for ongoing monitoring or to discuss treatment progress following discharge from a regular ED visit.

Virtual emergency departments are valuable for a variety of reasons. They provide access to emergency medical care for individuals who may be geographically distant from a physical emergency room or have difficulty reaching one due to mobility issues, transportation problems, or other barriers. Virtual care can significantly reduce waiting times compared to traditional emergency rooms, where patients often face long queues and delays. They enable resource optimisation. By handling less severe cases virtually, physical emergency rooms can allocate their resources more efficiently to patients in critical conditions. They also can facilitate a better response to pandemics. Virtual emergency departments proved vital during COVID-19 as they enabled healthcare providers to evaluate and treat patients while minimising the risk of virus transmission [7].

It's important to note that virtual emergency departments are not suitable for all medical emergencies. Some conditions require physical examinations, diagnostic tests, and immediate in-person interventions. Given the concerns around potentially missing something in the absence of a physical examination, clinicians may take a more cautious approach and have a low threshold for sending someone into the actual ED. Ultimately however virtual emergency departments are a valuable addition to the healthcare landscape, offering an alternative and convenient way for patients to receive timely medical attention while alleviating the burden on physical emergency facilities.

In terms of how it works in practice, a great example is the Victorian Virtual Emergency Department (VVED), which is 'a public health service designed to treat non-life-threatening emergencies', the first of its kind in Australia. The FAQ's below indicate how patients might optimally use the service and explains the process (Box 6.1).

Box 6.1 Summary of Virtual ED FAQ's
When should I call the Virtual Emergency Department?
Please call only if you have a non-life-threatening health emergency.
What is considered a non-life-threatening emergency?

Mild Respiratory Illness	Pain	Abdominal	Cardiovascular
Asthma	Abdominal	Nausea and/or	Palpitations
COPD	Limb	vomiting	Hypertension
Mild breathing problem:	Back	Diarrhoea	
Bronchiolitis/croup	Headache	Constipation	
Influenza		Urinary tract	
COVID-19		infections	

Neurological	Non-critical injury	Infection	Chronic conditions
Mild head injury Seizure Dizziness or fainting	Non-complex fracture Lacerations and skin tears Minor burns Soft tissue	Fever Skin or wound Urinary Respiratory	Diabetes Back pain Cancer Dementia
Women's health	Skin, allergies, insect bites	Ear, nose, throat and eye	General
Early pregnancy bleed Menstrual issues Early mastitis	Rash Oedema Insect sting Spider bite	Foreign body ear nose or eye Epistaxis Suspected tonsillitis	Falls or mobility concerns Wound dressings Abnormal pathology results

Can I talk to a doctor or nurse via phone?

No, we only do video consultations, as it improves the ability to assess your condition. You will need to use a device with a camera (mobile phone, PC, laptop or tablet). The camera must be turned on, and the patient must be awake to be triaged virtually.

How long will I need to wait online before I see a doctor or a nurse?

Wait times will fluctuate based on how many callers are online. However, on average, it is expected that you will be seen by an emergency doctor or nurse within 30 minutes.

When should I call an ambulance?

Please call an ambulance for life-threatening conditions. Examples include shortness of breath, severe chest pain, weakness down one side of the body. If you think you have a life-threatening condition, please contact Triple Zero (000) urgently.

Will I be speaking to a trained doctor?

All staff working for the virtual ED are fully qualified to deliver emergency care.

We have a team of emergency physicians, paediatric emergency physicians, paediatricians, general practitioners, medical registrars, nurses, and nurse practitioners ready to help.

What can I expect at my virtual ED visit?

The doctor or nurse practitioner will talk to you about your concerns. Depending on your needs, the doctor or nurse practitioner may suggest the following next steps:

- Sending a prescription to your pharmacy
- Making an appointment with a specialist doctor or clinic
- Ask you to see a family doctor or visit another Urgent Care Centre
- Ask you to go to your nearest Emergency Department for an in-person visit
  Nothing further, if your need can be addressed through the virtual visit

Other countries have taken similar initiatives. OTN is the Ontario Telemedicine Network, the virtual care division of Ontario Health (an agency created by the Government of Ontario with a mandate *to 'connect and coordinate our province's health care system to help ensure that Ontarians receive the best possible care'*) and has been working closely with its Cancer Care Ontario unit and Hospital partners to support two key facets of emergency care remotely: clinical assessment and treatment for non-life-threatening concerns [8]. The potential upsides for the local population and the health service are considerable. Patients seeking medical care or advice and who may be considering a trip to an ED, for instance, can log on to a Hospital webpage that includes ED information and use a live link to initiate a virtual visit from their own device, similar to the VVED example above.

The Ontario Health Portal Services available via the Virtual Front Door

Team-Managed Virtual Care

- eVisit: See your Doctor Virtually
- Indigenous services
- French language services
- Manage your COPD
- Manage Heart Failure
- Retinal screening for Diabetics
- Get Specialist Advice without the wait
- Virtual Palliative Care programme

Self-Managed Virtual Care

- Bounceback: Mental Health Coaching
- Problem Gambling Support
- Track Immunization Records

Via this digital front door an individual could be assessed in one of three ways:

- Through direct contact with an attending physician.
- Triaged remotely by either an actual nurse (using a tool like eCTAS—the electronic Canadian Triage and Acuity Scale) or
- An artificial-intelligence platform, such as a chatbot using sophisticated algorithms, that pre-screens them before connecting them with a clinician.

After triage, that same patient can then be placed in a virtual waiting room to see an available physician based on their acuity score or sent a scheduled time via text or email for a video or audio consultation. Prescriptions and lab tests can be ordered when appropriate—or, if necessary, the patient could be redirected to an in-person emergency department or an appointment with a primary care provider or urgent treatment centre.

Early evidence is supportive, research has shown that virtual care saves time, improves access, and can be easy to use. In a Canadian survey in May 2020, those who connected with their doctor virtually during COVID-19 reported a 91%

satisfaction rate with 46% indicating a preference toward a virtual visit as the first point of contact with their Doctor [9].

> *"I feel stronger about it, now that I see that people are calling in. They have trust in the care that we're giving. Some people are calling just to get reassurance that they're OK to stay at home. Some people are calling to get treatment over the virtual emergency care platform... we're providing successful care and people are pleased with the care they're receiving. So, we should be doing it"*—Canadian ED Physician

The Benefits of Virtual Emergency Care

There are multiple advantages to shifting more of the ED workload online and freeing up capacity for the more acute and life-threatening conditions that need to be seen face to face. Like virtual primary care, it is far more convenient, and it breaks down problems around accessibility, especially for people with mobility problems or who live in remote regions where normal ED facilities may be many hours travel away.

Reduced Waiting Times One of the most significant advantages of virtual emergency care is the elimination of long waiting times. Patients can remain in their own homes and connect with healthcare professionals almost instantly, resulting in quicker diagnoses and treatment plans.

Resource Optimisation By diverting non-critical cases to virtual platforms, physical emergency rooms can allocate resources more efficiently to patients who require in-person care. This optimises the use of healthcare resources and can lead to cost savings and more balances staff scheduling.

Continuity of Care Virtual emergency care ensures continuity of care by enabling follow-up consultations and monitoring after the initial virtual encounter. This is particularly beneficial for patients with conditions that might necessitate several repeat visits.

Pandemic Preparedness Virtual emergency care proved invaluable during the COVID-19 pandemic by allowing healthcare providers to safely evaluate and treat patients while minimising the risk of viral transmission.

Better Patient Experience and Satisfaction Not having to come into an Emergency Department has multiple advantages. It's more comforting and less anxiety inducing to be in your own home. The fact that a patient can have that first consultation without having to worry about transport will aid those who are less mobile, or less financially able to make their way to a hospital.

The use of video consultations upfront makes it possible for patients to have the first part of their emergency department journey undertaken at home. Often this can result in an altered journey to the standard wait for assessment in the ED. For example, a patient with a possible fractured ankle could be sent for a scan first, then go to an urgent treatment centre rather than the emergency department. A patient with an uncomplicated high blood pressure could be sent straight to the rapid access Cardiology clinic instead. For patients who do need to have an ED visit the senior clinician can often arrange for the correct diagnostic investigations, for example a CT scan, to be taken before the patient comes to the ED, saving the patient waiting and triage time which also helps reduce congestion in the ED environment. Evaluating HCP's can also arrange for immediate referral straight to the right speciality such as Gynaecology rather than needing to come to the ED at all.

These improvements can only be fully realised if the surrounding health service infrastructure can be organised in such a way as to respond. Therefore, careful resource planning and organisation across an integrated care network is often felt to be the best approach rather than individual elements of the health and social care services working in disparate siloes.

Limitations of the Virtual ED

There are of course some downsides to the virtual ED model so it is important to be aware of these and discuss so that they can be countered. These limitations could potentially impact the range and quality of care that could be provided, there are also implications for clinical safety, risk, governance and liability. It won't be long before we start to see legal test cases around medical negligence relating to virtual care provision.

Lack of Physical Examination Virtual emergency care relies on remote assessments, which may not allow healthcare providers to perform a thorough physical examination. Physical touch and in-person evaluation are often essential for diagnosing certain medical conditions accurately.

Limited Diagnostic Capabilities While virtual consultations can provide valuable information, they cannot replace the diagnostic capabilities of in-person healthcare settings. Some medical conditions require physical examinations or diagnostic tests that can't be conducted virtually. Providers must carefully evaluate which cases are suitable for virtual care. There are numerous diagnostic tests, such as X-rays, CT scans, and laboratory tests, that require specialised equipment that is not available during virtual consultations and minimal tests, or data gathering can be performed remotely unless a patient has kit such as a blood pressure machine or a pulse oximeter at home with them already. Although technology is advancing as we have seen with the GoodSam example in which smartphone cameras can pick up on some physiological measurements remotely.

Emergency Procedures Life-threatening emergencies, such as severe trauma, cardiac arrest, or certain surgical emergencies, require immediate interventions that can only be performed in a physical emergency room. Virtual care cannot replace the need for immediate in-person medical attention in such cases. However, in the future we may see devices such as portable defibrillators available for home use, and if a drug or piece of equipment needs to be provided, instructions for synthesising it could be sent directly to the domestic 3D printer. The focus however of most of the virtual ED models that we have discussed so far however emphasise that a great deal of the cases presenting to the emergency department are not acutal emergencies in the truest sense of the word. The systems that we are keen to elaborate on are those in which the non-emergencies are diverted elsewhere or dealt with remotely and this subsequently frees up the ED clinicians to crack open people's chest, re-inflate their lungs and restart their hearts.

Lack of Hands-On Care In some situations, patients may require hands-on care, such as wound management, sutures, or the administration of intravenous medications. Virtual care cannot provide these services. We're still a long way from home medical robots.

Limited Scope of Medication Prescribing While healthcare providers can prescribe medications during virtual consultations, there may be limitations on prescribing certain controlled substances or medications that require in-person monitoring, such as a cardiac drug or the first dose of an antibiotic. For safety, patients will need to come to a healthcare facility with the right supervision in place for many emergency treatments (which could be a day case unit or a UTC). Not everyone's carer or family member will be skilled enough (or happy to) deliver an intra-muscular injection.

Privacy and Security Concerns Telemedicine involves the transmission of sensitive patient information over digital networks. Protecting patient data and ensuring the privacy of virtual consultations is crucial, and there can be concerns related to data breaches or security issues with telemedicine platforms. Protecting patient data and ensuring the privacy of virtual consultations is a significant concern. Robust cybersecurity measures will be essential to maintain trust in virtual emergency care and comply with healthcare regulations like HIPAA in the United States.

Licensing and Jurisdictional Issues Healthcare licensing and regulations can vary by state or country, which can create challenges when providing virtual emergency care across different jurisdictions. Imagine a UK based GMC registered Doctor providing urgent patient management to someone in another country and some form of negligence or failure of care happening. Would they be liable for legal action in both their home country and the one in which the recipient was based? We're still in the early days of understanding how international law will handle such matters and it's likely that the costs of medical indemnity insurance could prove prohibitive to medical practitioners wanting to provide a service to those overseas. Clear guidelines and licensing requirements are needed to ensure quality and safety of care.

Reimbursement and Payment Models Establishing clear and consistent reimbursement policies for telemedicine services is an ongoing challenge. In some regions, reimbursement rates may be lower than in-person visits, making it less financially sustainable for healthcare providers.

Communication Challenges Effective communication is essential in emergency situations, and there may be limitations in conveying information and instructions through virtual means, especially in cases where patients have hearing impairments or language barriers. Following on from this is the problem of technological literacy—not all patients are comfortable or proficient in using digital technology for healthcare interactions. Healthcare providers may need to offer support and guidance to patients who are less tech-savvy in order to avoid digital exclusion (more on this in Chap. 12).

Information Siloes Delivering care across different organisations can be fraught with problems because of obtaining access to the right medical information for a patient. If clinicians are to work virtually successfully then they need unencumbered data access through interoperable systems. Something which is not always easy or forthcoming in many health services and especially important in an immediate emergency scenario.

Loss of the Personal Touch Although it is convenient and swift, virtual care may lack the personal touch and bedside manner that patients often value in healthcare interactions. This is especially relevant at times of urgent need and sudden deterioration. The time when you want a kind and considerate, friendly Doctor to hold your hand, look you in the eye and reassure you. Building trust and rapport can be far more challenging in a virtual setting. Maintaining empathy and effective communication is a challenge that providers must attend to because the risk is that this is seen as less essential in the context of high demands and high throughput systems.

It's important therefore to recognise that virtual emergency care is not a one-size-fits-all solution. While it can be effective for certain types of medical issues and emergencies, it is not a substitute for traditional in-person emergency care in cases of severe trauma, critical conditions, or situations that require immediate physical intervention. Healthcare providers, policy makers, clinicians and patients should carefully assess whether virtual care is appropriate for a given situation and be prepared to transition to in-person care when necessary. As telemedicine continues to evolve, efforts to expand access, enhance privacy and security, and refine regulatory frameworks will be essential to maximise its benefits while mitigating potential risks.

The Future of Virtual Emergency Care

Virtual care solutions promise to not only improve the patient experience but also tend to be relatively inexpensive to acquire and can be used in ways that tend to reduce cost or improve efficiency. This is hopefully a "win win." Better experience at lower cost and hassle.

Some of the key enablers in advancing the uptake and utility of telemedicine and the virtual ED concept include widespread adoption and acceptance of new technologies, improved audio-visual quality and internet connectivity (we may in future see greater use of virtual reality or augmented reality devices which will improve the quality of interactions), increasingly sophisticated remote monitoring devices (that can not only track a change in a patients physiological variables, that would alert the wearer to a deterioration, and be linked to a smart response system that would seek to correct the problem whilst medical assistance is being sought (examples of such systems include automated implantable cardiac defibrillators, which give the heart a shock if it goes into an abnormal rhythm, or a bi-hormonal pump system linked to a continuous glucose monitor that can adaptively control a person's blood glucose level).

Virtual care will become the "front door" to care for the majority of scenarios. It helps patients know who their provider teams are and to understand the resources available. It makes it easy to know where to go and how to connect for care. It adds convenience and will reduce Hospital use. The 'front door' engages patients by easily linking them to the right care providers and parts of the health services. Moreover, virtual care also provides a whole new array of tools for providers that can be offered to patients in an integrated care model.

Such approaches and experience may also be useful for governments and non-profit organisations to provide humanitarian support to other parts of the world. Telemedicine is being used in global health initiatives to provide healthcare services to remote and underserved regions around the world, including telemedicine supported clinics and disaster response. The future of virtual emergency care holds tremendous promise. Its ability to provide rapid access to medical professionals, reduce waiting times, and optimise resource allocation will transform emergency care delivery. Advancements in artificial intelligence (AI) and remote monitoring devices are set to enhance diagnostic accuracy and treatment recommendations. As technology advances and healthcare providers adapt, virtual emergency care will bridge the gap between patients and critical medical services. It is likely that a synergy between virtual and in-person healthcare will emerge. Combining the strengths of both approaches can create a comprehensive emergency care system that caters to a diverse range of patient needs.

References

1. Centers for Disease Control and Prevention. Emergency department visits. https://www.cdc. gov/nchs/fastats/emergency-department.htm
2. Cambridge and Peterborough Clinical Commissioning Group. The BIG conversation 27 September 2019 to 20 December 2019. End of conversation report. https://democracy. peterborough.gov.uk/documents/s41035/Item%206.%20Annex%201%20-%20BIG%20 Conversation%20report%20on%20feedback.pdf?txtonly=1
3. GoodSAM. www.goodsamapp.org
4. Smith CM, Lall R, Fothergill R, Spaight R, Perkins GD. The effect of the GoodSAM volunteer first-responder app on survival to hospital discharge following out-of-hospital cardiac arrest. Eur Heart J Acute Cardiovasc Care. 2022;11(1):20–31. https://doi.org/10.1093/ehjacc/ zuab103.
5. Linderoth G, Lippert F, Østergaard D, et al. Live video from bystanders' smartphones to medical dispatchers in real emergencies. BMC Emerg Med. 2021;21(1):101. https://doi. org/10.1186/s12873-021-00493-5.
6. NHS England. Transformation of urgent and emergency care: models of care and measurement. https://www.england.nhs.uk/wp-content/uploads/2020/12/transformation-of-urgent-and-emergency-care-models-of-care-and-measurement.pdf
7. Shuldiner J, Srinivasan D, Hall JN, May CR, Desveaux L. Implementing a virtual emergency department: qualitative study using the normalization process theory. JMIR Hum Factors. 2022;9(3):e39430. https://doi.org/10.2196/39430.
8. Canada Health Infoway. Virtual visits in British Columbia: 2015 patient survey and physician interview study. Ottawa, ON: Canada Health Infoway; 2016 Jul 25. https://www. infoway-inforoute.ca/en/component/edocman/resources/reports/3105-virtual-visits-in-british-columbia-2015-patient-survey-and-physician-interview-study. Accessed 23 Aug 2022.
9. Canadian Medical Association (CMA). What Canadians think about virtual care. CMA. 2020 May. https://www.cma.ca/sites/default/files/pdf/virtual-care/cma-virtual-care-public-poll-june-2020-e.pdf. Accessed 23 Aug 2022.

Further Reading

Agency for Healthcare Research and Quality. Most frequent reasons for emergency department visits. https://hcup-us.ahrq.gov/reports/statbriefs/sb286-ED-Frequent-Conditions-2018.pdf

Chapter 7
Proactive Care

Abstract Prevention, it is often said, is better than cure. In this new era, it makes sense that health services take advantage of new technologies, digital solutions and the power of data analysis to identify and target people who are at-risk of developing health related problems well in advance of them becoming problematic. Such technologies can be scaled to inform approaches to population health management and develop interventions that have wide scale impacts. Most would agree that disease prevention offers the greatest yield for population health and is amenable to a variety of digital health interventions via mobile and online applications, clinical kiosks and electronic patient portals. However, identifying return on investment and value for money can be large barriers to implementation, so good evidence is needed.

Keywords Preventative medicine · Preventive care · Remote monitoring · Personalisation · Patient empowerment · Proactive management · Risk factors · Public health · Population health · Wearables

What Is Proactive Care?

Healthcare is evolving, driven by both patients and healthcare providers, to move from a reactive approach to a proactive one. Proactive care using technology aims to prevent illness, manage chronic conditions, and optimise overall health through early prompt detection and continuous monitoring. In this chapter, we explore how technology is playing a pivotal role in transforming healthcare from a disease-centric model to one that is patient-centric, preventive, and predictive. If we can stop people becoming unwell at an early stage, or even prevent illness altogether then there is significant potential to alleviate major burdens on both individuals and wider society. 'Proactive care' is an approach that emphasises disease prevention through prompt intervention, modifying risk factors, developing tailored health plans, and deploying clever forms of monitoring. It contrasts with the traditional, reactive model of medical care, which mainly focuses on treating diseases and their symptoms, addressing health issues after they have already manifested. Key elements of proactive care include;

Prevention Preventative measures to reduce the risk of illness developing, for instance vaccinations (e.g. Polio has almost been obliterated from the world due to a prolonged, world-wide prevention programme), screenings, lifestyle modifications, and education on healthy behaviours.

New Zealand looked set to become the first country in the world to effectively ban smoking. Passing an anti-smoking bill in Parliament which bans the sale of tobacco products to anyone born after the 1st of January 2009. The ban was aimed at preventing future generations from taking up smoking and is part of a wider government push to make the country "smoke free". It would be accompanied by a slew of other measures to make smoking less affordable and accessible, including dramatically reducing the legal amount of nicotine in tobacco products and forcing them to be sold only through specialty tobacco stores, rather than corner stores and supermarkets. The country has also increased funding for health services and campaigns and rolled out quitting services specifically for Māori and Pacific communities. Subsequently the proposed ban was overturned, but surprisingly the UK Government looks like it is set to follow this positive approach, in order to 'protect the next generation'.

Early Detection Before symptoms become severe or irreversible. Regular checkups, health assessments, and diagnostic tests are essential components of early detection. Health screening for breast cancer using mammography in women over a certain age is a proven way of picking up malignant disease at a stage early enough for treatment to be successful. The elements that make up an effective screening programme are recognised to be;

- **The condition**—should be an important health problem as judged by its frequency and/or severity. The epidemiology, incidence, prevalence and natural history of the condition should be understood, including its development from latent to declared disease and there should be robust evidence about the association between the risk or disease marker and serious or treatable disease.
- **Acceptable test**—this should be a simple, safe, precise and validated. The test, from sample collection to delivery of results, should be acceptable to the target population i.e. not too traumatic, onerous or harmful. There should be an agreed policy on the further diagnostic investigation of individuals with a positive test result and on the choices available to those individuals.
- **Intervention that can do something**—there should be an effective intervention for patients identified through screening, with evidence that intervention at an early enough pre-symptomatic phase leads to better outcomes for the screened individual compared with usual (or no) care. Evidence relating to the wider benefits of screening, for example those relating to family members, should be taken into account where available.
- **The opportunity cost** of the screening programme (including testing, diagnosis and treatment, administration, training and quality assurance) - should be eco-

nomically balanced in relation to expenditure on medical care as a whole (value for money).

Personalisation Everyone has a differing risk profile and being able to personalise preventive measures is increasingly important, especially in the context of genomics. Proactive care may include recommendations for diet, exercise, medication, and other interventions based on an individual's personal risk, their family history and genetic makeup. Healthcare providers can tailor care plans to each individual's unique health needs and risk factors.

Continuous Monitoring Ongoing surveillance of an individual's health status. This can be achieved through health checks, regular follow-up appointments, remote monitoring devices, and health tracking tools. Various technologies can be incorporated into our environment to track our daily activities and wellbeing and it won't be long until they are built into the fabric of our cars, phones, homes and surrounds.

Patient Engagement Ensuring that people are actively engaged in their decisions about their healthcare and that they are encouraged to take ownership of their health allows greater respect for people's autonomy. Shared decision-making together with health education empowers individuals to make informed (and better) choices as they become more 'activated'. Lifestyle counselling, smoking cessation support and weight management have all been shown to have proven benefits and many of these could be delivered by remote or automated means such as the 'MyDiabetesMyWay' mHealth app or the Florence intelligent messaging service (which is a way of providing continuous, automated clinical conversations via text messaging).

Chronic Disease Management For people with long term illnesses such as heart disease, proactive care focuses on effective management (to optimise the health of the individual as much as possible) and monitoring e.g. daily blood pressure checks, to reduce the risk of the development of complications (eye disease, erectile dysfunction, kidney failure) and to help maintain quality of life.

Data-driven Decision Making Health systems and healthcare providers are able to use health information data to assess risk factors, track progress and make informed decisions about treatment and interventions, for example monitoring the rate of decline in kidney function in a patient or population of patients with diabetes over time (as shown in the graph in Fig. 7.1 below). Technology plays a significant role in data collection and analysis.

Focus on Wellness As well as detecting illness, proactive care needs to focus on promoting overall wellbeing and holistically consider the individual, taking into account lifestyle factors, mental health and the social determinants of health that contribute to a person's overall performance status, such as their postcode or their socio-economic status.

Efficient Resource Allocation By preventing disease and addressing health issues early, there is potential for a more efficient shift in the utilisation of healthcare resources (to non-preventable conditions), lower overall costs and ultimately better health outcomes.

It seems obvious but proactive care, emphasises disease prevention, early intervention, and ongoing health maintenance. Technology is increasingly becoming instrumental in facilitating the enablement of proactive care. Such technologies include wearable devices and sensors, patient portals and education platforms, telemedicine systems to enable remote consultations and increased accessibility to screening programmes. Tools such as wearables provide both individuals and health providers with lots of data and insights, facilitating early intervention and bespoke care plans. If you look at the early results from Apple, around the use of their smart watch technology, to detect a common cardiac abnormality called Atrial Fibrillation (AF) then it's easy to understand how useful such technologies are and the impact that they could have. Research published in the Journal of Cardiovascular Physiology showed that the Apple Watch has a high specificity for AF detection and can successfully be used for screening [2].

In a similar way, another piece of recent research from Liverpool in the UK targeted supermarket shoppers by installing a cardiac rhythm detecting device in the

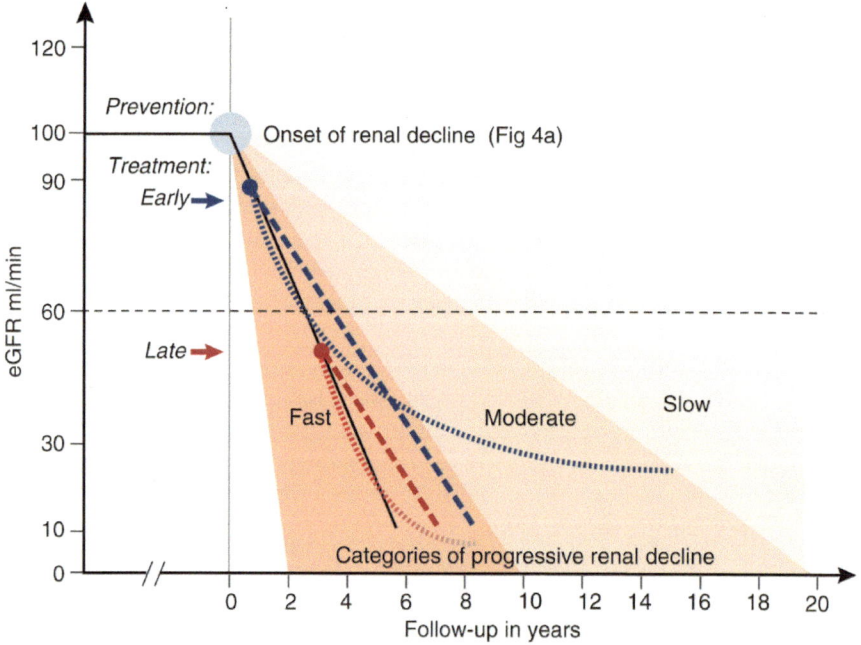

Fig. 7.1 Graph to show categories of declining kidney function over time and the outcomes of early versus late intervention. Reprinted from Krolewski et al. (2017) [1], with permission from Elsevier

handles of shopping trolleys (Fig. 7.2) [3]. Ten trolleys with a sensor in the handle—similar to those on gym exercise machines—were placed across four supermarkets. They managed to pick up 39 new cases of AF in previously unaware individuals over the course of 2 months. The handle sensors can identify cardiac arrythmias and this triggers the in-store pharmacist to undertake a manual pulse measurement and a static sensor reading to confirm the measurement. They can then offer a direct Cardiology referral. The implications of this opportunistic screening both for the health of those people and wider society is huge.

This study shows the potential of taking health checks to the masses without disrupting daily routines.—Professor Ian Jones [3]

A recent winner of the 'Ig Nobel' prize for public health went to Seung-min Park from South Korea, for the development of the Stanford smart toilet [4]. This clever device uses various technologies (including urine dipstick test strips and a computer vision system) to monitor human waste for signs of disease. This is an exceptionally sensible idea given that for millennia physicians have used excretia in order to diagnose diseases. Diabetes mellitus for example is characterised by very sweet tasting urine (due to excess glucose levels), whilst at the other end of the spectrum Diabetes insipidus produces foul tasting insipid urine. Bowel cancer, one of the big killers in the western world (contributed to by our awful diets) commonly causes small traces of blood in the faeces (often not perceptible to the naked eye). Imagine being screened for this every time you go to the bathroom and any abnormalities caught well before substantial problems and distress occur. Such technologies can be integrated into existing toilets and when they go into production may only cost around $300–600 to install. What if more than one person uses the same toilet I hear you ask. Well thankfully, it also has an anal-print sensor as part of its system in order to identify the user.

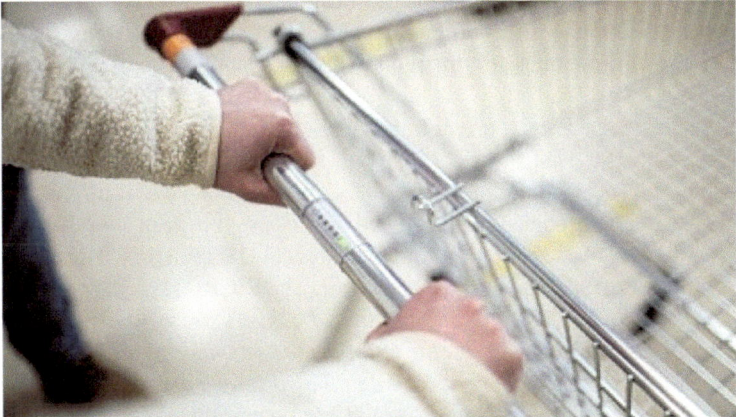

Fig. 7.2 Shopping trolley used to detect Atrial Fibrillation. Image Source: Jones et al. (2022) [3]. This article is an open access article distributed under the terms and conditions of the Creative Commons Attribution (CC BY) license (https://creativecommons.org/licenses/by/4.0/)

Ultimately the goal of proactive care is to improve health outcomes, enhance quality of life and reduce the burden of disease on society by addressing health problems proactively, (using technology is beneficial because it can automatically pick up on abnormal health information), rather than waiting for them to escalate to more serious or costly levels. It aligns with the principles of preventive medicine and population health management, aiming to keep individuals and communities healthier in the long term.

What Are Modifiable Risk Factors?

These are factors which can contribute to the development of a disease that are *"To a greater or lesser extent under the control of the individual"*, says the World Cancer Research Fund [5]. They involve people's lifestyles and include elements such as smoking, drinking alcohol, UV radiation/sun exposure, eating a healthy diet, including appropriate levels of fibre, fruit and vegetables and avoiding excess meat, partaking in safe sexual activities, undertaking physical exercise on a regular basis and not being overweight or obese. The wrong balance of these will lead to illness and a higher chance of death.

54% of bowel cancers are deemed preventable because they are linked to a lack of fibre, intake of processed meat or being overweight or obese. And almost one in four of the 61,500 new cases of breast cancer in the UK every year are also deemed preventable because they involve excess weight or alcohol [6]. It has been estimated by Frontier Economics that annually in the UK, 184,000 people will be diagnosed with some form of preventable cancer (such as skin cancer or bowel cancer) and that the ultimate costs of this to the economy will be around £78 billion pounds (which includes costs on families and carers as well as social services), the equivalent of 3.5% of GDP [6]. Worldwide levels of obesity are at 13% according to the World Health Organisation (with 39% of adults being overweight) which represents a huge risk for the development of malignant diseases and chronic illnesses such as Diabetes [7].

It's calculated that with current trends in the UK, the number of avoidable cancer diagnoses is due to rise from 184,000 to 226,000 a year by 2040 because of population changes. Over the intervening years, 3.7 million people will be diagnosed who would have not have otherwise developed the disease if it wasn't for the four known main risk factors—smoking, drinking, obesity and UV radiation. Those cases combined will cost the UK economy £1.26tn [6]. The WCRF says: *"When these [risk] factors alone are considered, around 40% of cancers are considered preventable. This means that if everyone was able to follow the recommendations related to each of the above factors, 40% of cancers would be prevented at a population level"* [5]. In short, four in every ten cancers would not occur and this 40% figure is fairly consistent across developed countries.

Research reported in the journal *BMJ* Oncology found that the number of under-50s being diagnosed with cancer worldwide had risen by 79% between 1990 and 2019 [8]. The authors from Zhejiang University School of Medicine, Hangzhou in China, said obesity, physical inactivity, alcohol and smoking were likely to help explain the surge, alongside other factors such as environmental pollution.

But it's not just these 'lifestyle-related' diseases that are preventable, a whole host of conditions based on demographics, social determinants, biological characteristics, postcodes, genetics and other risk factors can potentially be picked up early and something done about them. Unfortunately, this does not happen to the extent that it needs to.

What Are the Barriers to Proactive Care?

In an ideal world, it would be the status quo that the right level of disease screening and preventive care is undertaken, much of it on an automated basis, alongside simple nudges that support people to make better choices and allow them to have the best information on which to which make informed decisions about lifestyles. This doesn't happen to the extent that it could.

Screening and surveillance systems have to be very focused and there is so much temptation and ignorance around healthy behaviours that it can be difficult to make a meaningful impact. While proactive healthcare can lead to better outcomes and reduced healthcare costs in the long run, there remain several barriers and blockers that can hinder its adoption and effectiveness.

The limiting factors include lack of awareness, many people are not aware of the importance of proactive healthcare or the availability of preventive measures. This can lead to neglecting self-care behaviours or failing to attend screening programmes. Public health campaigns tell us that smoking is harmful, that being obese can cause cancer and that we should all be eating five portions of fruit and vegetables per day, but such messages struggle to penetrate our conscious awareness and they can be easy to dismiss or ignore.

In many countries, there is unequal access to health services, or failure of provision [9]. People without access to affordable healthcare may not be able to access preventative measures. Even when health insurance is available, high deductibles and co-payments can deter people from seeking proactive care (especially in the context of otherwise feeling well).

Other factors include time constraints—we're all leading busy lives and it is difficult to prioritise health checks, screening activities and healthy behaviours. Taking time off work or finding childcare for appointments can be challenging. Issues within the healthcare system, such as long wait times for appointments, limited access to specialists, and fragmented care, can discourage individuals from seeking healthcare proactively. In some regions, there may be limited resources for screening and prevention, including healthcare facilities and trained healthcare professionals to undertake the required work.

Health literacy is also highly relevant, many people simply do not know about the risks that they face and what could be done as preventative measures, this includes understanding medical recommendations, knowing what the warning signs of ill health to look for are, managing medications e.g. to lower cholesterol, and making informed decisions about health, such as safe levels of alcohol intake or the best approaches to weight loss. Following on from this, cultural beliefs and language barriers can affect people's willingness to seek preventive care and their ability to communicate effectively with healthcare providers. Then we have denial, fear of receiving bad news or the stigma associated with certain health conditions which can all discourage individuals from seeking help or getting checked out. In the age of the internet and social media there is a maelstrom of misinformation—this can lead to misconceptions and misguided decisions about one's health and if this is allied with a perception of invincibility, or the *'what the hell effect'*, this can prevent people from taking proactive steps to manage their health.

Studies in the US have shown that 8.6 hours per working day are required for a clinician to fully satisfy the US Preventive Services Taskforce preventive care recommendations for their patients [10]. However, the competing demands of managing existing acute and chronic disease in the context of an ageing population saturated with complex multi-morbidity, makes it near impossible for the right preventive care to be delivered. There are several interventions which already exist to try and surmount this problem including the 'patient-centred' medical home, increasing use of community health workers, and integration of primary care services with public health [11]. These all seek to alleviate the burden on hard working clinicians but given that there is a dynamic evolution of health technologies it seems timely and appropriate to use digital solutions to take on much of this workload.

Public Health, Public Policy

Given the interest in this area, and recent announcements of large-scale investments in AI, it is unsurprising that better use of data and technology are central themes for Government and health service's prevention plans. These need to look at providing targeted support, personalised care and lifestyle support and greater protection against future threats. It's thought that new technologies such as genomics and AI will enable new prevention models and if there is better data sharing between different elements of the health service a new wave of intelligent public health can allow greater patient engagement and more tailored health interventions. For example, the UK Government's green paper 'Advancing our health: Prevention in the 2020s' sets out five challenges that need to be addressed if they are to harness the full potential of digital solutions [12];

1. Balancing interventions that reduce individual susceptibility vs. interventions that tackle the underlying causes of disease.
2. Balancing universal interventions against targeted approaches.
3. Making prevention services accessible to those who need them most.
4. Closing the evidence gap between prediction and prevention

5. Balancing investment in novel solutions against funding tried and tested solutions.

It is hoped that new, 'smarter' approaches to prevention will help address entrenched problems (such as health inequalities) and worrying trends (such as the stalled improvements in life expectancy). However, if real progress is going to be made in improving the public's health, history tells us that some fundamental tensions in public health policy and practice need to be addressed. For instance, achieving the best balance between support mechanisms for risk reduction at an individual level, in contrast to more broad spectrum population level interventions. Data and technology will enable a more tailored approach but it is important that the big picture determinants of health (environmental, educational and socio-economic) are not forgotten.

One major research review by KJ Thomas Craig and colleagues from the IBM Watson Research and Evaluation group in Massachusetts has looked specifically into whether digital health interventions (such as telemedicine, clinical decision support systems and mHealth) can help reduce health inequities, such as those faced by people from minority ethnic groups, lower socio-economic classes, and people in some rural and urban settings [13]. They reviewed a large body of research work undertaken in the field of digital health in the context of cardiovascular disease between 2008 and 2020. Interestingly they found that the use of newer digital health technologies significantly improved health outcomes (both clinical and patient reported) and standards of healthcare delivery (accessibility, quality, care utilisation) in populations that were disproportionately affected by heart disease in the majority of studies analysed. This provides good evidence that digital health interventions can help to mitigate some of the traditional problems and negative social factors. It's encouraging that digital solutions such as telehealth may have the capacity to reach patients that traditional forms of health care do not. However, a lot more still needs to be done to tackle the underlying causes of the causes of illness and disease in our society.

To overcome the barriers and blockers to better population health management, healthcare systems, policymakers, and communities must work together to raise awareness, improve access, reduce costs, and provide education about the importance of proactive healthcare. This is the approach that has intermittently been taken for many years and has only been partially successful. To what extent can technology do more?

How Can Technology Support Proactive Care?

Before the emergence of the coronavirus and the subsequent pandemic in 2020, the health and care system had a poor track record in adopting digital technologies at scale. However, in response to the lockdown restrictions the health care system rapidly implemented new tools, many technology-based, to allow health care to be delivered in new and interesting ways, as we've seen throughout this book. The approach to using digital tools in health care provision is similarly undergoing a substantial and rapid shift.

Digital health interventions can support preventive care on many fronts, for example coordinating the timely receipt of vaccinations to at risk populations (winter flu vaccinations for the elderly and vulnerable), the identification and processing of at-risk individuals for screening programmes and ensuring that those with pre-existing chronic medical conditions, such as Diabetes, undergo routine monitoring and treatment optimisation through algorithm based approaches. This all relies on the connection between primary care databases, public health disease registries, care management programmes and electronic patient records, so that linked data becomes meaningful and provides actionable insights.

There are numerous technologies that can be used in health prevention across various aspects of healthcare.

Mobile Health (mHealth) Apps Data amassed by Pew Research indicates that around five billion people worldwide have mobile devices, more than half of which are smartphones [14]. The technologies within these devices have improved iteratively and it is now possible to have access to computing power that could steer a spacecraft, GPS, a high-speed internet connection and high-quality imaging capabilities in the palm of our hands, alongside a host of sensors for health-relevant data (e.g., movement and location tracking), plus a touch-screen interface. Yet the use of smartphones in health and care still falls short of the potential to create and monitor personalised digital biomarkers that combine with new data sources to improve prevention, treatment and help people make sustained behaviour changes.

App stores already feature thousands of health and wellbeing apps, encompassing everything from diet diaries and mindfulness guidance to period trackers and musculoskeletal rehabilitation support. However, the uptake by the health and care system has been patchy due to a range of issues including cost, quality, evidence, clinician knowledge, confidence and skills, and integration into pathways. Efforts to curate the best quality apps, for example, in the NHS App Library, have had little success in making the use of apps for health mainstream. A growing number of apps now focus on a direct-to-consumer approach largely focusing on health information, self-care or monitoring. Apps have also been developed to provide digitally enabled interventions (these are known as **digital therapeutics**). These provide reminders for medications, track physical activity, and offer personalised health plans for example. Patients can set goals, monitor their progress, and receive guidance tailored to their specific health needs. Mobile apps offer a wide range of health prevention tools, including:

- Diet and nutrition apps that provide personalised meal plans and track calorie intake.
- Fitness apps that offer exercise routines, monitor physical activity, and set fitness goals.
- Medication reminders to ensure individuals take their medications as prescribed.

- Mental health apps that provide stress reduction techniques and emotional support.

Digital therapeutics are health or social care interventions delivered either entirely or mostly through a device (smartphone, tablet, virtual-reality or augmented-reality system, or a laptop). They effectively embed clinical practice and therapy into a digital form. At a minimum, these interventions combine the provision of clinically curated information on a health condition with advice and techniques for dealing with that condition. For example, a clinician could prescribe a person with a history of depression or anxiety an app that incorporates, for example, breathing exercises, meditation, or cognitive behavioural therapy (CBT). Such an app could give regular support alongside self-care to help the person overcome episodes of depression without needing to seek in-person help and wait for an appointment.

Whether fully automated or blended with supervision (or coaching), the therapy offered can be adjusted to the needs of the specific user. Digital therapeutics are often cited as a solution to help manage long-term conditions that call for behaviour changes or to prevent diseases in the long run.

The purpose of such apps is to provide feedback on one's health status, facilitate monitoring of a particular condition, or to stimulate behaviour change. It is thought that their use is an effective strategy for improving health promotion behaviours in the general population. In one systematic review by Lee and colleagues from Yonsei University in Korea, it was found that health outcomes were shown to be better for app-users when compared with non-users [15]. Most app-driven digital health interventions (DHIs) included in Lee's study were patient-facing and focused on helping to better involve patients in their care. Given that app based proactive care is becoming increasing commonplace for a variety of health promoting behaviours (from dietary intake to step count to mindfulness), we can expect its coordinated utilisation by health services to increase in years to come.

However, app-driven DHIs are also capable of providing an overwhelming amount of data to providers. Balancing data collection features from apps by adding functionalities, such as thresholds triggering clinical alerts and feedback, designing patient-counselling suggestions based on gathered data, and pairing with timely contact is important to enhance the clinical relevance and quality of these tools. As the development and clinical adoption of app-driven DHIs continues to expand, rigorous investigation of their safety, efficacy, and value of them will be needed.

Social Media Monitoring As well as their potential use as a mechanism for promoting healthy living, smartphones are also a portal into the mire of social media (and social inattentiveness). Healthcare researchers can however use information harvested from micro-blogging platforms such as X, Threads and Bluesky, to monitor the spread of infectious diseases, including COVID and SARS and predict disease spread and activity. By scanning millions of online posts and searching for instances of the word 'flu' amongst other keywords, hashtags and geolocation data, it's possible to study disease trends and use social media as an effective disease monitoring tool. It can be far more up to date and accurate than traditional tools to follow an epidemic and serve as an early warning system for disease outbreaks.

There is also scope for community engagement and targeted public health messaging in affected areas via social media, as well as a role in the rapid identification and combatting of misinformation to limit the spread of false health theories.

At Home Diagnostics and Test Kits Home diagnostic tests can help individuals assess their risk factors for various conditions, such as heart disease or genetic predispositions to certain diseases. This works best if the equipment is cheap or free or can easily be utilised in conjunction with a smartphone. Results from at-home tests can in principle motivate individuals to make positive lifestyle changes, like adopting healthier diets, increasing physical activity, and quitting smoking.

Remote monitoring devices, such as blood pressure cuffs, glucose meters, and pulse oximeters, allow individuals to track their vital signs at home. Diagnostic devices often come with accompanying apps or platforms that allow users to upload, track and visualise their health data over time, providing insights into their health trends. These devices can be connected to healthcare providers' systems, enabling remote monitoring, detect abnormalities early and facilitate sooner intervention for several conditions. Some at-home tests, like colorectal cancer screening kits, allow for early detection of diseases, improving the chances of successful treatment. This type of technology can expedite access to healthcare in remote or underserved areas, or during pandemics, where getting to a healthcare facility can be challenging and helps to reduce exposure to contagious diseases. Overall, at-home diagnostics can support proactive care by giving individuals the tools they need to take charge of their health and well-being, leading to better health outcomes and a more patient-centred approach to healthcare.

Wearables/IoT Devices One of the pillars of proactive care is the use of wearable and Internet of Things (IoT) devices. These include fitness trackers, smartwatches, blood pressure monitors and glucose meters. These devices continuously collect and transmit vital health data to users and their healthcare providers. For instance, a patient with diabetes can monitor their blood glucose levels in real-time, and the data can be shared with their healthcare team, allowing for early intervention if levels become unstable. Wearable devices are increasingly valuable in preventive care because they provide continuous monitoring and real-time data about a person's health and lifestyle. They can detect irregularities in vital signs, sleep quality or notify users of potential health issues. Wearable systems are generally in direct contact with the wearer for long durations, generating large quantities of data on specific biometrics or behaviours. They can alert users to an abnormality in their pulse or blood pressure, detect a fall, remind people to take their medication, and recommend changes in activity levels based on personal patterns. Patients with congestive heart failure can have their weight and blood pressure data sent to their care team daily. Any sudden weight change can be an early indicator of worsening symptoms, prompting timely interventions.

Many large technology companies are positioning these devices as health or wellness devices, not medical devices—currently side-stepping regulatory requirements. They are even being developed to track and alert users about the onset of degenerative conditions such as Parkinson's or Alzheimer's disease. A user could have the level of medication in their blood regularly monitored according to a physician's plan and be reminded to administer their next dose when its level drops below a certain threshold. The Business Research Company states that, "*Intelligent wearable sensors promote the transformation of healthcare from a traditional hospital-centred model to a personal portable device-centred model*" [16]. More on this type of tech in the next chapter.

Artificial Intelligence AI is an umbrella term encompassing a number of different approaches where software replicates functions that have until recently been synonymous with human intelligence. This includes a wide spectrum of abilities such as visually identifying and classifying objects, converting speech to text and text to speech, etc. Although the use of AI or artificial intelligence is not new in healthcare, the development of this type of technology in healthcare has accelerated significantly in recent years. AI is beneficial in many ways, including developing new pharmaceuticals, triaging, and orientating patients, computer-assisted surgery, or improving diagnosis processes through virtual assistants. AI technologies are used to collect, analyse, and utilise data to automate specific recurring tasks and allow clinical teams to focus on tasks with higher value. AI-powered algorithms can analyse large datasets to identify health risks, predict disease outcomes, and recommend personalised preventive measures. This is especially important in the context of both preventative medicine but also population health management. When AI is combined with machine learning (a process in which computer systems can learn without being explicitly programmed) medical programmes can recognise patterns in data when exposed to new information. This will allow new insights into big datasets. The hope is that machine learning when applied to medical databases and demographic information will be able to identify clusters of health risks, detect early warning signs, predict future health outcomes, and recommend interventions—at a population level. In terms of population health analytics, healthcare organisations can use data tools to identify health trends, assess risk factors, and predict health outcomes for populations. This information guides management, resource allocation, and health promotion campaigns. Another use for data-driven technology could be to identify and target those who are not currently reached by prevention interventions. If initiatives can use linked data to target and monitor the impact of the health checks in marginalised groups, this could help reach the people who are currently missing out.

Several tech organisations are looking to harness machine learning techniques to provide diagnostic support to help improve disease detection and subsequent care delivery. For example, Deepmind has published research evaluating AI applied to breast cancer screening showing improved efficacy, and start-ups, such as Ultromics, are applying machine learning to improve speed and reduce variability in the diagnosis of cardiovascular disease from ultrasound images. In the future, machine learning tools will be able to quantitatively interpret images to create digital biomarkers that predict onset of disease. For example, the current EVAREST study is a multi-centre trial aiming to validate blood and imaging biomarkers, the first step to achieving diagnosis based on machine learning-powered digital biomarkers.

Genomic Testing and Personalised Medicine The first complete genome sequence of a living organism was produced in 1995, with the first human genome sequenced in 2003, costing approximately $2.7 billion over the course of a decade. Since then, the economics of genome sequencing has changed significantly. In 2003 it was commonly believed that a $1000 genome sequencing cost would unlock the ability to perform personalised medicine. With the cost now trending towards a few hundred of dollars this aim has been surpassed. Such advances in genomic sequencing technology enable the practice of precision medicine and allows individuals to undergo genetic testing to assess their risk of developing specific diseases. This information can inform personalised prevention plans, including tailored screening and lifestyle recommendations. If an individual does develop an illness with a genetic component, the genetic profile of their disease and knowledge of the likely response to treatment can be calculated and it should be possible to find out more about the effectiveness of medical interventions, such as prescribing drugs to treat a disease (pharmacogenomics).

Large Scale Research Smartphones and wearables are highly effective data collection devices, and they can record a lot of detail about people's lives. As well as tracking their own health status, people can also help researchers gather large amounts of real-world data on their activity, health problems and their determinants using their smartphones or wearables.

Open-source frameworks, including Apple's ResearchKit and ResearchStack for Android devices, have paved the way for the development of apps tailored for medical research. These systems have streamlined the process of transferring apps between platforms, making it easier to reach a wider audience. Specialised apps utilise surveys and consent forms to allow users to opt-in for research purposes. Additionally, they enable automatic collection of data from user devices, such as step counts and heart rate, in order to support data sharing efforts. Since 2015, these platforms have ignited a fresh method of studying diseases, resulting in numerous extensive opt-in studies. In 2016, for instance, over 4000 individuals willingly participated in a study on Parkinson's disease. Similarly, in 2018, more than 400,000 people enrolled in a study on atrial fibrillation, while in 2017, over 8000 individuals took part in an asthma study. More recently, 250 individuals are currently being identified to participate as 'citizen scientists' in a study on adolescent arthritis [17].

The recruitment of a large number of participants within a relatively brief timeframe would not have been achievable without the utilisation of a digital application-based strategy. These research studies possess the ability to enhance our comprehension of how diseases change over time and the corresponding lived experience of individuals. Moreover, they've also enhanced and normalised the utilisation of smartphones and wearable devices as digital indicators for medical research. In the future, researchers will have the ability to establish individual benchmarks using this data, measure an individual's personal experiences, monitor their digital markers, enhance diagnosis, and accurately observe the progression of diseases and the effectiveness of treatments.

E-Health Education and Health Literacy Tools Online educational resources and health literacy tools can empower individuals to make informed health decisions. These digital resources are accessible and user-friendly, supporting health prevention efforts. When used effectively they have the potential to empower individuals and play a crucial role in promoting proactive health management and wellness and subsequently reduce the burden of preventable diseases in our society.

People are the common driving force behind all technologies. The internet and smart devices have facilitated connections that can bring communities together. These connections allow individuals with shared identities and common interests in health and disease to share knowledge, coping strategies, and support one another. Additionally, these technologies provide a platform for tracking health data and managing conditions. Social networks for health, such as MedHelp, PatientsLikeMe, and HealthUnlocked, have played a significant role in this regard. In fact, data from PatientsLikeMe has contributed to published studies in various clinical areas, including depression, ALS, and multiple sclerosis.

By empowering individuals, healthcare providers, and public health organisations, these technologies enable early identification of health risks, promotion of healthier behaviours, and disease prevention. This approach is more empowering than government health campaigns or the paternalistic approach of traditional medicine because it allows for openness and agency, supported by a sense of community. Technology improves access to information, enabling individuals to make better decisions about their health and gain more control and knowledge about their wellbeing. It is important to note that the technologies mentioned here are just a few examples, and there are many others that have the potential to transform health and care. However, further evidence is needed to fully understand their costs and benefits and ensure they deliver on their promise.

What Are the Implications of Radically Improved Population Health Management and Proactive Care?

Improving population health has far-reaching implications that extend beyond individual well-being to impact society, healthcare systems, economies, and overall quality of life. These implications are both broad and significant, making population health improvement a critical goal for governments, healthcare organisations, and communities.

Reduced Healthcare Costs Effective population health management can lead to cost savings in healthcare systems. By preventing or managing chronic conditions, reducing emergency room visits, and promoting healthier lifestyles, healthcare costs can be minimised. This can result in a more efficient allocation of healthcare resources and a reduced financial burden on individuals and governments.

Enhanced Productivity A healthier population is arguably a more productive one. When individuals are healthier, they are more likely to work and be engaged in their communities. Reduced absenteeism and improved productivity can have positive effects on economic growth and overall prosperity.

Increased Life Expectancy Similarly lower mortality rates mean that individuals have more years of productive life, contributing to economic growth and reducing the societal burden of early death.

Improved Quality of Life Better population health objectively leads to an improved quality of life for individuals. Reduced disability, better mental health, and increased overall well-being contribute to happier and more fulfilling lives. Healthier communities often exhibit greater social cohesion and community engagement. When people feel well and secure, they are more likely to participate in community activities and support each other.

Health Equity Population health improvement initiatives often address health disparities and social determinants of health. This can lead to greater health equity, ensuring that all members of society, regardless of socioeconomic status, have the opportunity to attain their highest levels of health. Population health improvement initiatives aim to reduce healthcare disparities among different demographic groups. This promotes social justice and equality, leading to a fairer and more inclusive society.

Resilience to Pandemics and Health Emergencies A population with improved health is better equipped to respond to pandemics and health emergencies. Strong public health infrastructure and proactive health promotion can mitigate the impact of infectious diseases and other health crises.

Healthcare System Sustainability and Long-Term Planning By focusing on prevention and early intervention, healthcare systems can become more sustainable in the long term. Managing chronic conditions early can reduce the burden on healthcare facilities and resources. Population health improvement necessitates long-term planning and sustainable policies. This forward-looking approach encourages governments and organisations to invest in the health and well-being of future generations.

Innovation and Research Opportunities Improving population health generates opportunities for research and innovation in healthcare and public health. New technologies, treatments, and interventions can emerge from efforts to address health challenges.

In summary, improving population health has wide-ranging positive implications that extend from individual health and well-being to economic prosperity, social equity, and global cooperation. Ultimately, it reduces preventable suffering, alleviates the physical and emotional pain that individuals and families experience due to health-related issues, fostering a more compassionate and caring society. Technology therefore has the potential to address health disparities by improving access to healthcare services, enhancing healthcare delivery, promoting health equity, and addressing the social determinants of health that contribute to disparities.

Challenges and Ethical Considerations

While technology holds great promise in supporting proactive care, it also brings challenges and ethical considerations. These include data privacy and security, ensuring equitable access to technology, and the potential for over-reliance on algorithms in medical decision-making. Privacy concerns, data security, health disparities, and ensuring equitable access to technology are critical issues that must be addressed in the implementation of digital large scale health management strategies.

Using Data to Target High-Need Groups Data-driven technologies have the potential to identify and target individuals who are currently not benefiting from prevention interventions. By utilising linked data, initiatives can specifically focus on marginalised groups and monitor the impact of health checks, thereby reaching those who are currently being overlooked. However, there is a significant issue with the data systems that facilitate this process. These systems often reflect the structural inequalities present in our society. For instance, many risk-prediction advancements rely on genetic datasets that have historically excluded numerous populations. The majority of participants in genetic studies are of European ancestry, accounting for 79% of the total [18]. Although efforts are being made to address this disparity, current tests may still exclude certain groups, which poses a problem in our increasingly diverse societies. Furthermore, data often contains biases that perpetuate existing problems, and poorly designed algorithms can reinforce biases in risk assessment processes. Non-Caucasian groups are frequently underrepresented in data sources, which increases the risk of excluding individuals. Once the assessment of those at highest risk has been conducted, the subsequent challenge for public health is to translate this knowledge into effective strategies for preventing illness. While understanding risk is crucial, the history of tobacco control demonstrates that utilising this information to improve population health can be unexpectedly challenging. Currently, there exists a gap between prediction and prevention evidence.

The Issue of Age Digital technologies, such as wearable devices, smartphone applications, and health websites, have the potential to contribute to the promotion of health and prevention of diseases among the general population. Specifically, younger individuals who are more educated and better off tend to utilise digital technologies for promoting a healthy lifestyle and also report a higher level of perceived digital health literacy.

Interestingly, there is limited knowledge about the specific needs of older individuals when it comes to utilising digital technologies for promoting a healthy lifestyle in the digitalised world [19]. Despite being considered nondigital natives and facing various barriers in using digital technologies, these technologies can actually facilitate healthy aging by providing access to health information and healthcare services. For instance, older individuals can only benefit from digital health offerings if they have access to appropriate technological devices like tablets or smartphones. The initial adoption of such technologies depends on their acceptance by the target population. Therefore, digital technologies designed for older individuals should be user-friendly and clearly communicate their usefulness. Additionally, continuous engagement with these technologies is crucial for their effective utilisation. This requires adequate digital health literacy and human support to operate and potentially gain benefits from digital technologies. In general, the development of suitable digital technologies for healthy aging in older individuals necessitates co-creation and feedback from the target population. Furthermore, evaluating the cost-effectiveness and user outcomes in the context of health promotion and disease prevention is essential for a better understanding of how digital technologies function and their potential impact.

Other barriers for the roll out of digital solutions are, language, cultural and social issues, education, and health literacy and importantly the so-called digital divide, in which those who are likely to be most in need of proactive healthcare provision—the at-risk individuals—are the least likely to have access to smart devices and the internet.

Ways of overcoming some of these barriers include other forms of technological support. Cultural competencies and language access—technology can support language access services, making healthcare information and services available in multiple languages. Additionally, cultural competency training programs for healthcare providers can be delivered online to improve care for diverse patient populations. Automated text messaging and telephonic outreach can be used to remind patients of appointments, medication schedules, and preventive screenings. These reminders can aim to improve healthcare adherence in underserved populations. Education and health literacy—online educational resources and health literacy tools can empower individuals to make informed health decisions. Technology can provide easy access to health information in user-friendly formats, aiding understanding and decision-making. 'Digital Equity Initiatives' comprise efforts to bridge the digital divide, such as providing affordable internet access and devices to underserved communities, with the goal of ensuring that technology-based health solutions are accessible to all.

Gayle Stephens, writing back in 1965, highlighted a crucial point that seems to have been overlooked with the widespread adoption of technology. She pointed out that *"One of the paradoxes of our time is that the healing relationship seems most in jeopardy at a time when we need it most"*. Stephens referred to *"forces which threaten to de-personalise the meeting of a doctor and patient"* [20]. This paradox still persists in today's age, where technology is often viewed as a distraction, rather than a tool that improves patient care, and we must continue to be mindful of this in our implementation efforts.

Summary

Prevention should be the cornerstone of modern healthcare. Advancements in technology have the potential to revolutionise the way we approach prevention and help keep people healthy and free from illness. Indeed, this is already happening in patches. But there are also dangers, such as the potential for novel solutions to increase health inequalities, and there are real opportunity costs. Digital solutions are enhancing the practice of population health management, enabling healthcare organisations to proactively address the health needs of communities and wider patient populations. By leveraging data analytics, telehealth, care coordination, and patient engagement tools, population health care can become more efficient, effective, and patient-centred. The future of healthcare relies on the continuous integration of digital solutions to drive positive health outcomes for diverse populations, reduce health disparities, and promote well-being on a large scale. In order to achieve this, health services must establish the best balance across various domains.

1. Emphasising interventions that will have the greatest impact on population health by addressing broader determinants of health, rather than just individual susceptibility.
2. Alignment between universal interventions and targeted interventions. While there may be benefits to targeting existing services, such as screening, the costs and benefits must be carefully weighed and robustly evaluated.
3. Applying data and technology solutions in a way that reduces health inequalities and benefits those who are most in need. This includes explicitly addressing the impact of new solutions on health inequalities and considering the barriers that certain groups face in accessing preventive services.
4. Addressing the evidence gap between prediction and prevention. Simply calculating risk in more detail does not automatically lead to more effective prevention or improved health. Robust research and evaluation are necessary to bridge this evidence gap.
5. Balancing investment in novel technological solutions with the ongoing need for investment or reinvestment in proven prevention methods. Effective use of modelling methods and rigorous, rapid evaluation can ensure that limited resources are not wasted on solutions that have little or no impact on population health.

These challenges must be tackled for new data and technology solutions to truly make a difference in population health. To fully capitalise on the opportunities, government's visions of utilising new data and technology for public health must go beyond personalisation and consider the broader potential for improving the health of the public.

References

1. Krolewski AS, Skupien J, Rossing P, Warram JH. Fast renal decline to end-stage renal disease: an unrecognized feature of nephropathy in diabetes. Kidney Int. 2017;91(6):1300–11. https://doi.org/10.1016/j.kint.2016.10.046.

2. Wasserlauf J, Vogel K, Whisler C, et al. Accuracy of the Apple watch for detection of AF: a multicenter experience. J Cardiovasc Electrophysiol. 2023;34:1103–7. https://doi.org/10.1111/jce.15892.

3. Jones ID, Lane DA, Lotto RR, et al. Supermarket/hypermarket opportunistic screening for atrial fibrillation (SHOPS-AF): a mixed methods feasibility study protocol. J Pers Med. 2022;12(4):578. https://doi.org/10.3390/jpm12040578.

4. Park SM, Won DD, Lee BJ, et al. A mountable toilet system for personalized health monitoring via the analysis of excreta. Nat Biomed Eng. 2020;4(6):624–35. https://doi.org/10.1038/s41551-020-0534-9.

5. World Cancer Research Fund. Preventing cancer, saving lives. https://www.wcrf-uk.org/

6. Frontier Economics. The societal and economic costs of preventable cancers in the UK, 2023. https://www.frontier-economics.com/media/edwnhnlc/frontier-economics-the-societal-and-economic-costs-of-preventable-cancers-in-the-uk.pdf

7. World Health Organisation. Obesity and overweight fact sheet. https://www.who.int/news-room/fact-sheets/detail/obesity-and-overweight

8. Zhao J, Xu L, Sun J, et al. Global trends in incidence, death, burden and risk factors of early-onset cancer from 1990 to 2019. BMJ Oncol. 2023;2:e000049. https://doi.org/10.1136/bmjonc-2023-000049.

9. European Commission. Inequalities in access to healthcare, a study of national policies. https://ec.europa.eu/social/BlobServlet?docId=20339&langId=en

10. Privett N, Guerrier S. Estimation of the time needed to deliver the 2020 USPSTF preventive care recommendations in primary care. Am J Public Health. 2021;111(1):145–9.

11. Ferrante JM, Balasubramanian BA, Hudson SV, Crabtree BF. Principles of the patient-centered medical home and preventive services delivery. Ann Fam Med. 2010;8(2):108–16.

12. UK Government. Advancing our health: prevention in the 2020's. https://www.gov.uk/government/consultations/advancing-our-health-prevention-in-the-2020s/advancing-our-health-prevention-in-the-2020s-consultation-document

13. Thomas Craig KJ, Morgan LC, Chen C-H, et al. Systematic review of context-aware digital behavior change interventions to improve health. Transl Behav Med. 2021;11(5):1037–48.

14. Pew Research Centre. Mobile fact sheet. https://www.pewresearch.org/internet/fact-sheet/mobile/

15. Lee M, Lee H, Kim Y, et al. Mobile app-based health promotion programs: a systematic review of the literature. Int J Environ Res Public Health. 2018;15(12):2838. https://doi.org/10.3390/ijerph15122838.

16. TBRC Business Research PVT LTD. Research company's wireless healthcare global market report 2022. https://www.globenewswire.com/news-release/2022/04/05/2416930/0/en/Wearable-Devices-Are-Gaining-Popularity-In-The-Wireless-Healthcare-Market-Fueled-By-Rising-Demand-For-Self-Monitoring-As-Per-The-Business-Research-Company-s-Wireless-Healthcare-Glo.html

17. Walls TA, Coria A, Forkus SR. Citizen health science: foundations of a new data science arena. Int J Popul Data Sci. 2019;4(1):1074. https://doi.org/10.23889/ijpds.v4i1.1074.

18. Martin AR, Kanai M, Kamatani Y, Okada Y, Neale BM, Daly MJ. Clinical use of current polygenic risk scores may exacerbate health disparities. Nat Genet. 2019;51:584–91. https://doi.org/10.1038/s41588-019-0379-x.

19. Ienca M, Schneble C, Kressig RW, Wangmo T. Digital health interventions for healthy ageing: a qualitative user evaluation and ethical assessment. BMC Geriatr. 2021;21(1):412. https://doi.org/10.1186/s12877-021-02338-z.

20. Stephens GG. The personal touch: the physician as healer in modern society. J Kans Med Soc. 1965;66:237–9.

Further Reading

Bauer UE, Briss PA, Goodman RA, Bowman BA. Prevention of chronic disease in the 21st century: elimination of the leading preventable causes of premature death and disability in the USA. Lancet. 2014;384(9937):45–52.

De Santis KK, Jahnel T, Sina E, Wienert J, Zeeb H. Digitization and health in Germany: cross-sectional nationwide survey. JMIR Public Health Surveill. 2021;7(11):e32951. https://doi.org/10.2196/32951.

Kebede AS, Ozolins L, Holst H, Galvin K. The digital engagement of older people: systematic scoping review protocol. JMIR Res Protoc. 2021;10(7):e25616. https://doi.org/10.2196/25616.

McKinney SM, Sieniek M, Godbole V, et al. International evaluation of an AI system for breast cancer screening. Nature. 2020;577:89–94. https://doi.org/10.1038/s41586-019-1799-6.

Radcliffe Department of Medicine. About the EVAREST study. https://www.rdm.ox.ac.uk/about/our-clinical-facilities-and-mrc-units/cardiovascular-clinical-research-facility/evarest-1/about-evarest

Roland KB, Milliken EL, Rohan EA, et al. Use of community health workers and patient navigators to improve cancer outcomes among patients served by federally qualified health centers: a systematic literature review. Health Equity. 2017;1(1):61–76.

Thomas Craig KJ, Fusco N, Lindsley K, et al. Rapid review: identification of digital health interventions in atherosclerotic-related cardiovascular disease populations to address racial, ethnic, and socioeconomic health disparities. Cardiovasc Digit Health J. 2020;1(3):139–48. https://doi.org/10.1016/j.cvdhj.2020.11.001.

UK National Screening Committee. Criteria for a population screening programme. Updated September 2022. https://www.gov.uk/government/publications/evidence-review-criteria-national-screening-programmes/criteria-for-appraising-the-viability-effectiveness-and-appropriateness-of-a-screening-programme

Chapter 8
The Monitored Self

Abstract With the growth of smart devices, wearables and remote monitoring there is a major opportunity for individuals to learn more about themselves, their physiological variables and how things change with time, activity, emotions, strong coffee, and various external stimuli and stressors. This is not just for curiosity and narcissism, but it allows individuals a window into the inner workings of their own complex physiology, something that was never previously easily available. The benefit of such insights is bio-feedback—understanding how your own unique biological markers respond to the world. This in turns enables 'performance management' of the self. Controlling, adapting, changing and modifying inputs in order to achieve the right outputs or target goals from glucose stabilisation to weight loss, to blood pressure control and more. This is not just the realm of the dedicated ultra-athlete it's becoming an emerging reality for the masses.

Keywords Wearables · Remote monitoring · Proactive care · Internet of things · Sensors · Self-management · Patient engagement · Empowerment · Digital health solutions

What Do We Mean by the Monitored Self?

The term "monitored self" refers to the practice of individuals actively tracking and monitoring various aspects of their own health and well-being, using digital technologies and tools. It involves the use of devices, apps, wearables, and sensors to collect and analyse data related to one's physical and mental health, lifestyle, and behaviours (Fig. 8.1). The goal of the monitored self approach is to gain insights into one's health and make real (or near real) time, informed decisions to improve well-being, prevent health issues, or manage existing conditions.

Self-monitoring is not a new concept, it's been around for many years, often used to support habits and behaviour change, for example tracking food intake using a food diary, recording mood or symptoms of mental health over time, keeping a sleep journal or simply measuring progress towards a personal goal such as quitting

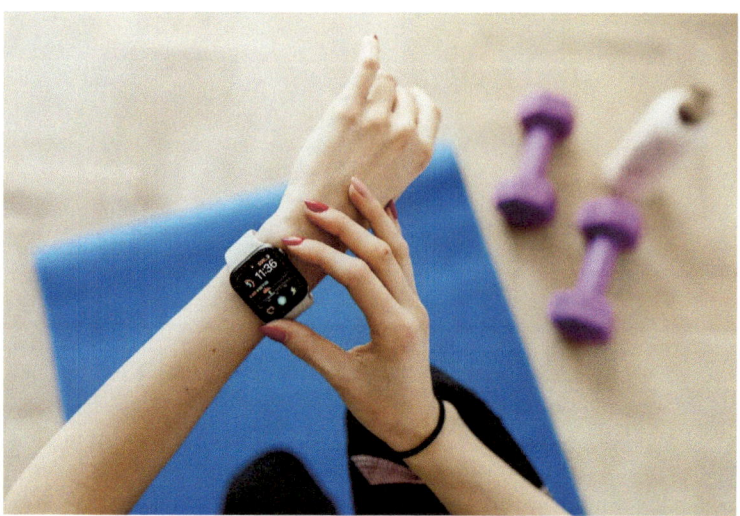

Fig. 8.1 Modern smart watch wearable monitor. Credit: Karolina Kaboompics. Image Source: Unmodified from Pexels.com (https://www.pexels.com/photo/anonymous-sportswoman-checking-smart-watch-and-sitting-on-mat-4498483/)

smoking. For it to be effective, the monitoring has to be frequent, consistent and accurate enough to capture a measurable change, honest (human beings often have a tendency to omit results that cast them in a bad light, such as a high blood glucose level after a takeout pizza) accurate, and meaningful. Given the rise in technologies which can capture increasingly detailed information about our metabolism and other body systems and the fact that this can be largely automated, this means that self-monitoring is becoming more accessible and impactful, and leads us towards the holy grail of patient engagement, shifting at-risk individuals from the contemplation stage of behaviour change into affirmative action.

An Overview of Technology Types

Wearable Devices These include wearable technologies such as smartwatches, fitness trackers, and health-monitoring devices that can track parameters like heart rate, step count, sleep patterns, and more. These devices provide continuous data collection and feedback to the user and are already widely available with a widening array of applications. Wearables are increasingly integrated with telehealth platforms, allowing users to share real-time health data with healthcare providers between in-person and during virtual visits.

Wearable Biofeedback Devices These devices provide biofeedback for stress reduction, anxiety management, and performance optimisation are gaining popular-

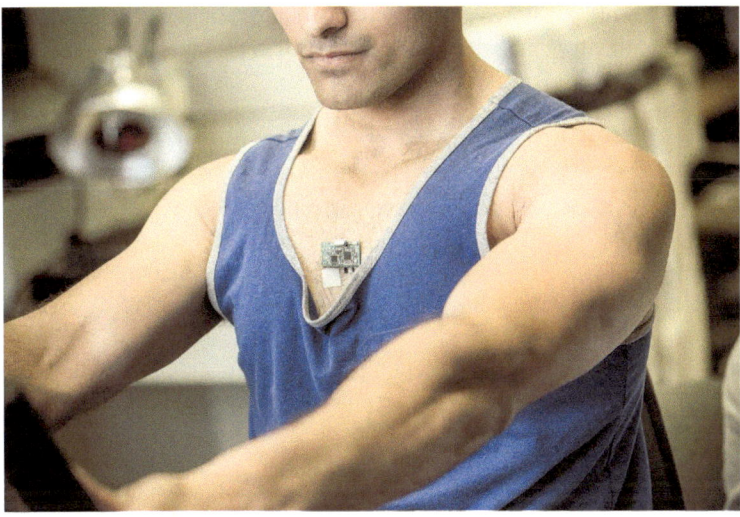

Fig. 8.2 The rise of biosensors. Image Source: UCSD Jacobs School of Engineering. (https://today.ucsd.edu/story/engineers_take_first_step_toward_flexible_wearable_tricoder_like_device). Reproduced with permission from Professor Amay Bandodkar

ity (Fig. 8.2). They often use factors such as heart rate variability (HRV) data to guide users in relaxation exercises. Devices like sensory wristbands can provide calming or stimulating sensory feedback to help manage symptoms of conditions like autism or dementia.

Wearable Smart Patches These slim devices adhere to the skin and can monitor various health metrics, including hydration, glucose levels, and medication adherence. They are discrete and comfortable for long-term wear. Smart (or biometric) tattoos are the next step. Devices which embed circuitry or electronic components, data stores and remote monitors under the skin to monitor and interact with the user's body. These tattoos can serve various purposes, including health monitoring, user authentication, or as a means of interfacing with digital devices.

Wearable Tech for Seniors Wearables designed specifically for seniors may include fall detection, medication reminders, medical alert devices to call for help in an emergency, and simplified interfaces for ease of use. Supportive functions might also include the use of GPS trackers, or smart clothing, so that carers can track the location of their loved ones if they have dementia or a tendency to wander off or set up geofencing. AI powered smart glasses can assist with tasks such as reading, navigation, or providing augmented reality guidance (Fig. 8.3).

Health and Wellness Apps Mobile applications allow users to log and track various health-related data, including diet, exercise, medication adherence, and mood.

Some apps also offer features like goal setting and reminders, but also data sharing (not just for with your clinical team but also with peers and family members).

Remote Monitoring Healthcare providers may remotely monitor patients' vital signs and health conditions, especially for individuals with chronic diseases (such as a continuous glucose monitor for a person living with Diabetes) or post-operative care needs. This allows for early intervention and reduces the need for frequent in-person visits. Advanced sensors can measure blood glucose levels, blood pressure, oxygen saturation, and more. They provide users with valuable health information and can alert them to potential issues.

Connected Home Devices Smart home devices can monitor indoor air quality, temperature, humidity, and other environmental factors that can impact health and comfort.

Data Analytics Data collected through these monitoring technologies can be analysed to identify trends, correlations, and anomalies. Users can gain insights into their health and well-being, potentially leading to lifestyle changes or better disease management.

Mental Health and Stress Management Wearables are incorporating features to monitor and manage stress levels, sleep quality, and mental health. Some devices

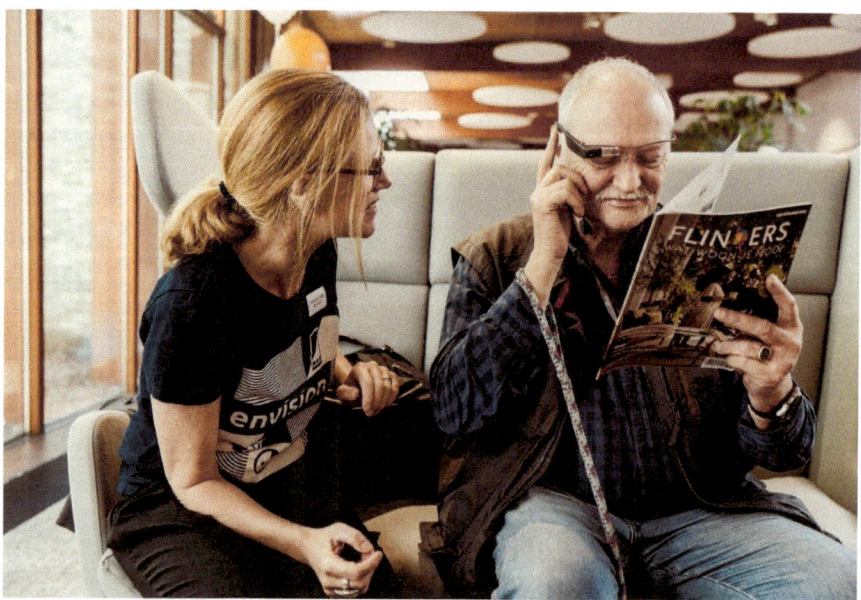

Fig. 8.3 Smartglasses to augment reality. Image Credit: Reproduced with permission from Envision (https://www.letsenvision.com/glasses)

Fig. 8.4 The Reflect Orb
biofeedback device. Image
Source: reproduced with
permission from Reflect
(https://www.meetreflect.
com/shop/)

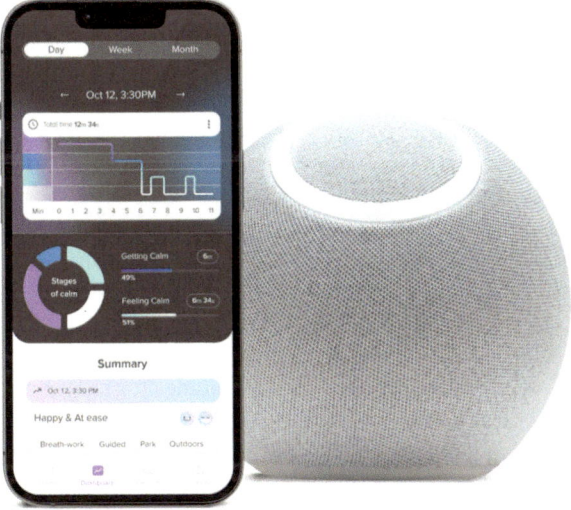

use biofeedback and guided meditation techniques to promote relaxation, such as
the Reflect Orb shown in Fig. 8.4 below which connects to an app and when held
uses HRV and electrodermal activity measurements to '*glow in different colours,
vibrate and guide you to a calmer state*'.

Personalised Health and Wellness Plans The data collected through the monitored self can be used to create personalised health and wellness plans, including
fitness routines, dietary recommendations, and stress management strategies.

These technology trends reflect the increasing integration of technology into
healthcare and the growing emphasis on personalised health and wellness as people
seek to take greater ownership of their health (or potentially an unhealthy obsession
for the worried well). As wearable health tech continues to advance, it has the potential to play a significant role in improving health outcomes and promoting proactive
health management. A scoping review by researchers Kang and Exworthy from the
University of Birmingham in 2022 showed that considerable findings in the literature suggest that wearables can empower individuals by assisting with diagnosis,
behaviour change, and self-monitoring [1]. However, greater adoption of wearables
and engagement with devices depends on various factors, including promotion and
support from providers to encourage uptake; increased short-term investment to
upskill healthcare staff, especially in the area of data analysis; and overcoming the
barriers to use, particularly by improving device accuracy.

Such approaches to monitoring do not always have to be highly active. Technology
can take on the burden of monitoring and allow people to get on with their lives.
Max Parmentier, the founder and chief executive of a novel start up called Birdie
explains, "*Birdie is a leader in home healthcare technology; we build digital tools
that help homecare businesses streamline their operations*". The inspiration for

Birdie came from recognising that for most people, the best place to grow older is at home—it's where we're healthier, happier and supported by our wider communities. *"The problem was that while social care is an industry that deserves best-in-class technology and continued investment, it had up to that point been largely left behind in the digital revolution. We knew the change had to come from within—so we decided to build the technology ourselves"*, says Max. A SaaS platform at its core, Birdie includes mobile apps for care professionals and family members, and a web app for homecare providers, all linked to in-home remote monitoring systems. For family members of the care recipient, updates from the app ensure they are kept in the loop around their loved one's care. For anyone that has worried about an elderly relative (which is many of us), this visibility and peace-of-mind is invaluable. The ultimate benefit of such monitoring technology is that it enables people to remain independent in their own homes for longer, without having to sell up and go into a nursing or care home with all the restrictions that this implies.

Max concludes *"We all know that the current social care system is broken, and in an ageing society this problem is only going to become more acute: we believe that through the power of intelligent technology we have the opportunity to transform how elderly care is delivered. In the years to come, we'll see Birdie bring to life a new vision of the 'circle of care', empowering care recipients to take control of their care journeys for truly person-centred care"*.

Selina's Story

Selina always wanted to be a gymnast. She trained from a young age, and her family based in Northern California, encouraged her ambitions, taking her to practice regularly and travelling to competitions at weekends. When Selina was 14 years old she started to lose a significant amount of weight, her periods stopped and she began to lose interest in what had previously been her obsession. Her parents were worried that she might be depressed or taking drugs, but there was a strong background family history of diabetes and one of her aunts who herself had type 1 diabetes, met Selina after not having seen her for some time and was shocked by the change in her appearance. *"I asked Selina was she peeing a lot"* recalls Marita, the aunt, *"as soon as she said yes, I knew that she had Diabetes. I used my glucometer to check her blood sugar and the reading came back 'HI', no number, it was off the charts"*.

When Selena was diagnosed with type 1 diabetes she had to be trained to use a finger prick blood glucose machine and test her blood sugars before and after every meal, when she got up in the morning and before going to bed at night. She had to learn how to inject herself with insulin and she had to write down her blood glucose readings in a little book that she then presented to her paediatrician or diabetes nurse on every clinic visit. Often, she would be criticised for not responding to a particularly high or low blood glucose value and it took her a long while to get the right balance of medication and relate this to her activity levels, her food intake, her menstrual cycle and her day-to-day performance.

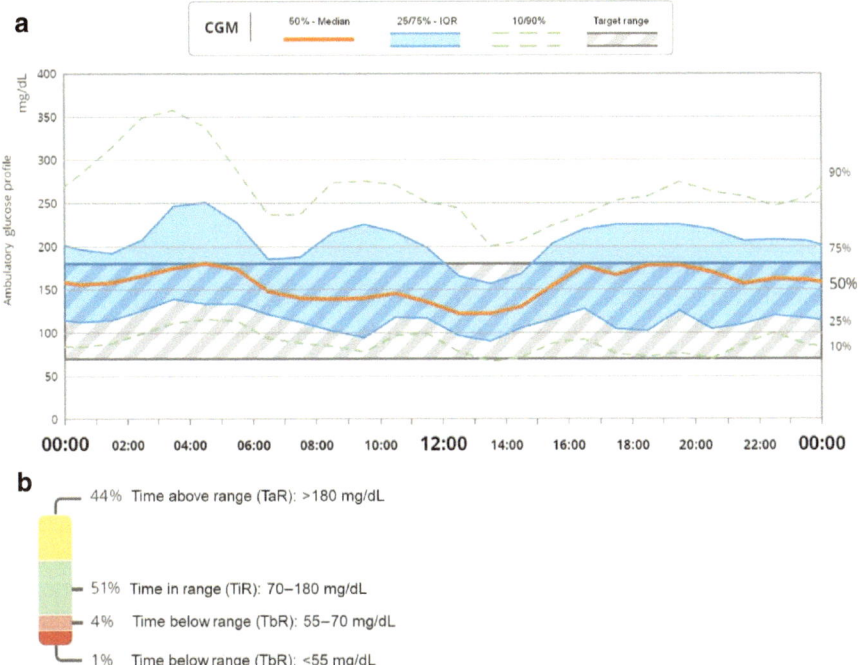

Fig. 8.5 Ambulatory glucose profile generated from a flash glucose monitor, supporting biofeedback. Image Source: Reproduced with permission from Guido Freckmann, graph generated with Dexcom CLARITY® software [2]. (**a**) represents the pattern of her glucose throughout a 24 hour period. (**b**) provides a breakdown of the time spent in each of the different glucose ranges

After 1 year she was she was given a combined blood glucose monitor and insulin pump system. The goal of these types of systems is to act as an 'artificial pancreas' to try and replicate the missing biological functions that happens in type 1 diabetes. Using the system helped to lessen her anxiety around self-management significantly (Fig. 8.5). She learnt to understand her blood glucose patterns better because the sensor gave her a read out on her smartphone.

Her weight recovered, her mood improved, she felt more in control and eventually returned to her love of gymnastics. She feels that the power that the monitoring system gave her set a free again and within 6 months she became a regional champion. Her mother brightly says that the monitoring system 'Gave us our daughter back'.

Communities

Many people (from fitness self-trackers, athletes and those with chronic medical conditions such as hypertension) are increasingly sharing their monitored self-data with groups of other like-minded individuals, who voluntarily collect and share personal health and wellness data. This is typically through online platforms, social networks, or specialised communities. These communities often have a common interest in health, fitness, wellness, or a specific medical condition. The shared data may include information such as fitness achievements, dietary habits, sleep patterns, medication adherence, and health metrics like HbA1c, heart rate and blood pressure.

Many of these communities exist on social media platforms, dedicated health and wellness apps, or websites specifically designed for data sharing and tracking. Popular platforms include Strava, Fitbit Community, MyFitnessPal, and various disease-specific forums and groups.

Some members share data for personal accountability, while others use it for motivation or to seek advice from peers. Some communities organise health challenges, competitions, or events that encourage members to reach specific goals or milestones. These challenges often include friendly competitions, awards, or recognition for achievements.

Groups may collectively analyse and interpret their shared data to gain insights into trends, correlations, or patterns related to their health or wellness. This collaborative approach can help individuals get advice from experienced peers and make more informed decisions about their well-being. In addition to data sharing, these communities often serve as platforms for exchanging knowledge and information related to health and wellness topics. Members can ask questions, share research findings, and provide guidance based on their experiences. Privacy and data security are essential considerations in these communities. Platforms allow users to control the level of data sharing and visibility to protect their privacy of their personal information.

Many monitored self-data sharing communities focus on fostering a positive and supportive environment, emphasising achievements and progress rather than negative aspects or setbacks. Some communities dedicated to specific medical conditions or health issues also serve as platforms for advocacy, raising awareness, and supporting research efforts related to those conditions. In some cases, healthcare professionals may actively participate in or provide guidance to these communities to ensure that the information shared aligns with evidence-based practices and safe health behaviours.

The benefits of such collective data sharing include peer support and motivation. Members can exchange tips, experiences, and encouragement, which can be motivating and helpful in achieving health and wellness goals (so long as such forums are well moderated—it's important for individuals to exercise caution and verify the accuracy of information they encounter).

What Are the Implications of the Monitored Self Approach?

Table 8.1 below summarises the advantages and disadvantages of taking such a detailed and proactive approach to self-care.

Table 8.1 Summary table of the impacts of the monitored self approach

Advantages	Disadvantages
Technology can make the day-to-day management of a medical condition easier for many	Technology can feel like a burden
Technology can help people living with a chronic disease manage their condition more effectively	There can be an overwhelming amount of data generated
Technology can reduce the risk of negative disease complications and outcomes	Technology is not always perfect or accurate
Technology can support people to reach their targets	Technology can break or fail
Data can be shared with healthcare professionals	Technology isn't a quick fix—it's important to manage people's expectations

The monitored self approach, which involves individuals actively tracking and monitoring various aspects of their own health and well-being using digital technologies and tools, offers several benefits.

Personalised Health Management Allows tailoring of individual's health and wellness strategies to their unique needs and goals. By collecting and analysing personal data, they can make informed decisions about their lifestyle, diet, exercise, and healthcare choices. Individuals who engage in the monitored self route often adopt healthier lifestyles, including better nutrition, increased physical activity, and reduced stress. Setting health goals, tracking progress, and sharing achievements with others can boost motivation and provide a sense of accountability.

Preventive Health Regular self monitoring helps individuals detect potential health issues early, enabling them to take preventive measures and make lifestyle changes to reduce the risk of chronic conditions and diseases if they are able to develop the right insights and connections. If individuals and healthcare providers identify deteriorations in health sooner, it enables timely interventions and hospital admission avoidance.

Empowerment Technology empowers individuals to take an active role in their health. They hopefully become more engaged, informed, and motivated to make positive changes and adhere to treatment plans. It reduces reliance on the medical profession and evens out the relationship. Greater engagement often involves seeking health information and education, leading to improved health literacy and better-informed decisions.

Improved Health Outcomes By tracking and managing their health, individuals can ideally set goals, achieve better health outcomes, manage chronic conditions more effectively, and reduce the risk of complications.

Cost Savings Preventing or managing health issues early can lead to cost savings in healthcare expenses by reducing the need for hospitalisations, medications, invasive treatments and the management of complications.

Data-Driven Decisions By providing individuals with actionable data to make decisions about their health and wellness it can be used to set and track progress towards health goals.

Medication Adherence Tracking medication schedules and adherence using digital tools can improve medication management and treatment efficacy.

Healthier Lifestyles Patient-Provider Collaboration—sharing monitored self-data with healthcare providers fosters better communication and relationships, allowing providers to offer more personalised care and guidance.

Improved Mental Health Using new technologies can help individuals better understand and manage their mental health by tracking mood, stress levels, and sleep patterns.

Research and Discovery Aggregated and anonymised self-monitoring data can contribute to research and the discovery of health trends, potentially leading to advancements in healthcare.

It's important to note that while the monitored self approach offers numerous benefits, individuals should use digital health tools and monitor their health responsibly. Privacy and data security considerations are crucial, and individuals should consult with healthcare professionals for guidance and interpretation of monitored data, especially for managing complex medical conditions or making significant health-related decisions.

There are some disadvantages and potential challenges that individuals (and healthcare providers who recommend such systems) should consider:

Data Accuracy and Reliability The accuracy and reliability of data collected through consumer-grade devices and apps can vary. Factors like sensor accuracy, device calibration, and user error may affect the quality of data and lead to erroneous results and actions. There was a delay with the approval of flash glucose monitoring devices becoming a valid measure of blood glucose levels before driving because of the lag between the 'true' blood glucose value and the interstitial fluid glucose values being picked up by the monitoring system. This means that if a person with diabetes' blood glucose value is on the way down prior to driving, they may be at risk of having a hypoglycaemic episode whilst in the car, having received false reassurance from their device that they were still in the normal range.

Data Overload Collecting a vast amount of health data can be overwhelming. Individuals may struggle to interpret and make sense of the data, leading to confusion or anxiety.

Data Privacy and Security Storing and sharing personal health data electronically carries privacy and security risks. Data breaches, unauthorised access, and misuse of health information are concerns [3]. Internet connected wearable devices and health apps can be vulnerable to cybersecurity threats, potentially exposing sensitive health data to hackers (see Fig. 8.6 below).

Health Anxiety Constant monitoring and access to health data may lead to health anxiety or hypochondria, where individuals become overly concerned about minor health fluctuations.

Dependency on Technology Some individuals may become overly reliant on technology for health monitoring, potentially neglecting other essential aspects of health, such as regular visits to healthcare providers.

Inaccurate Interpretation Misinterpreting health data or drawing incorrect conclusions from monitoring data can lead to unnecessary worry or inappropriate self-treatment. Some individuals may attempt to self-diagnose or self-treat based on monitoring data without consulting healthcare professionals, potentially leading to mismanagement of health issues.

Information Overload for Healthcare Providers Healthcare providers may receive large amounts of patient-generated health data, making it challenging to

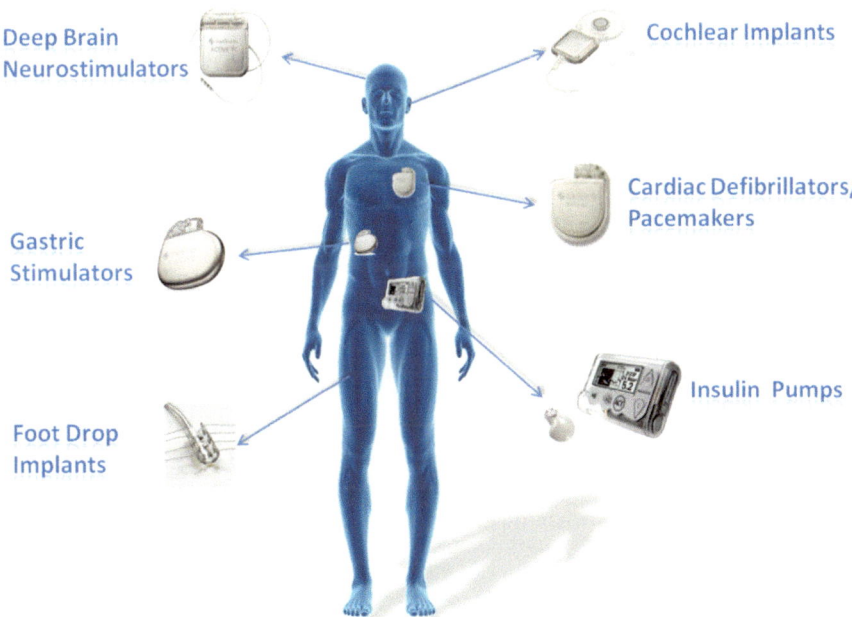

Fig. 8.6 Overview of current forms of implantable medical devices. Image Credit: reproduced with kind permissions from Haitham Hassannieh (https://groups.csail.mit.edu/netmit/IMDShield/)

integrate and interpret this data within their regular practice. Huge volumes of data are already coming through from cloud-linked flash glucose monitors and this is not quick and easy data to absorb, digest and synthesise before or during an out-patient consultation. Plus, the data often lacks clinical context, making it challenging for healthcare providers to assess its relevance and make informed decisions.

Device Cost High-quality wearable devices and health-monitoring equipment can be costly, making them inaccessible to some individuals.

Device Compatibility Compatibility issues may arise when individuals use multiple devices and apps from different manufacturers, leading to data fragmentation because of interoperability problems [4].

Regulatory Challenges The regulatory landscape for health apps and wearables is evolving, and not all devices and apps may meet the necessary standards for accuracy and safety.

Loss of the Personal Touch We come back to this important point, over-reliance on digital monitoring may diminish the personal touch and human connection in healthcare, which can be important for patient-provider relationships. This has been a recurrent theme throughout this book that technologies run the risk of detracting from traditional Doctor-Patient relationships.

To mitigate these disadvantages, individuals interested in the monitored self-approach should:

- Choose reputable and clinically validated devices and apps.
- Be mindful of data privacy settings and security measures.
- Seek guidance from healthcare professionals for interpreting and acting on monitoring data.
- Use monitoring data as a complement to, not a replacement for, regular healthcare check-ups.
- Avoid self-diagnosis and treatment without professional consultation.

Ultimately, the monitored self approach can be a valuable tool when used responsibly and in conjunction with expert medical advice and care. It empowers individuals to take an active role in their health management, make informed decisions, and detect potential health issues early. It can lead to improved health outcomes, better adherence to treatment plans, and a greater sense of control over one's well-being. However, it's essential to use these technologies responsibly, and to consult with healthcare professionals when making significant health-related decisions or interpreting monitoring data.

References

1. Kang HS, Exworthy M. Wearing the future-wearables to empower users to take greater responsibility for their health and care: scoping review. JMIR Mhealth Uhealth. 2022;10(7):e35684. https://doi.org/10.2196/35684.
2. Freckmann G. Basics and use of continuous glucose monitoring (CGM) in diabetes therapy. J Lab Med. 2020;44(2):71–9. https://doi.org/10.1515/labmed-2019-0189.
3. Wadhwa T. Yes, you can hack a pacemaker (and other medical devices too). Forbes 2012. https://www.forbes.com/sites/singularity/2012/12/06/yes-you-can-hack-a-pacemaker-and-other-medical-devices-too/
4. WHO. Medical devices: managing the mismatch: an outcome of the priority medical devices project. 2010. https://www.who.int/publications/i/item/9789241564045

Chapter 9
Spare Parts

Abstract Regenerative medicine is the process of creating living, functional tissues to repair or replace tissue or organ function lost due to damage, disease or congenital defects. This field holds the promise of fixing damaged tissues and organs in the human body by stimulating previously irreparable organs to heal themselves or to find a way to replace them entirely. This has the potential to solve the problem of the shortage of organs available for transplant as well as overcoming the risk of organ transplant rejection.

Such advances will progressively disrupt the concept of healthcare delivery in Hospitals by switching them from reactive repair shops struggling to combat the deterioration in the human body, to more of a surveillance based system, tracking changes in organ function over time and providing avoidance therapies based on stem cells and DNA manipulation, and secondly, as being a spare parts service, generating replacement human organs to order which can then be inserted, plumbed in and put to work. Such approaches will reform clinical practice and human behaviours in unimaginable ways.

Keywords Regenerative medicine · Artificial organs · Stem cells · Genetic engineering · Personalised medicine · Transplants · Incurable diseases

What Is Regenerative Medicine?

Management of human illness is largely based around trying to retard disease progress and the development of complications, or providing the body itself an opportunity to heal by ameliorating the impact of harms. As healthcare services increasingly take advantage of new technologies we will see a major paradigm shift in the way that hospitals work and the fundamental ways in which we think about medical care delivery. Regenerative medicine is the field of science in which living functional tissues can be created to repair or replace tissues or organ function which have been lost due to damage, disease, or congenital defects (Fig. 9.1). It holds the promise of stimulating previously irreparable organs to heal themselves or find a way to replace

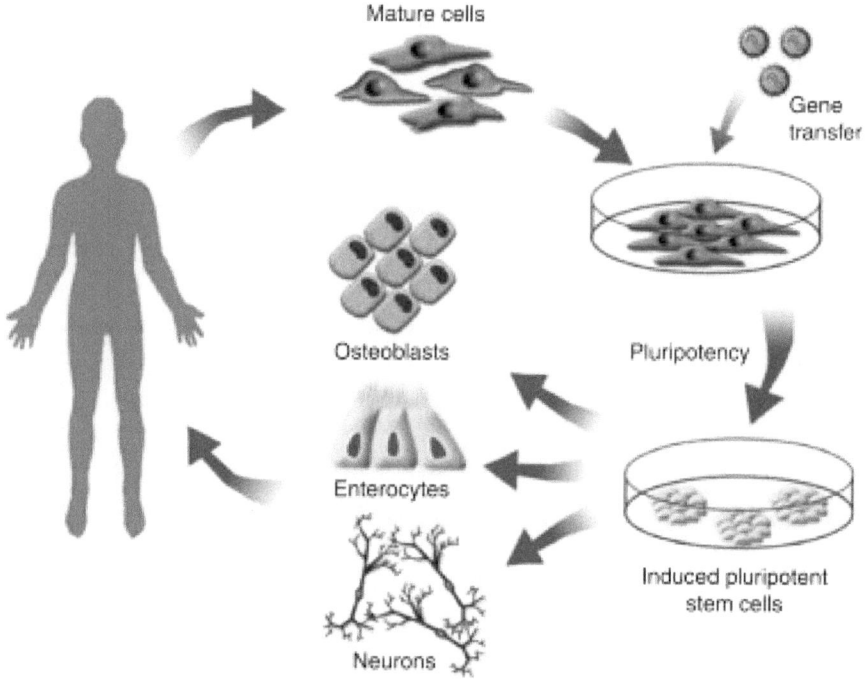

Mature cells

Gene
transfer

Osteoblasts

Pluripotency

Enterocytes

Induced pluripotent
stem cells

Neurons

Fig. 9.1 Overview of stem cell production for use in regenerative medicine. With permissions from Chagastelles and Nardi (2011) [1]

them entirely by regenerating damaged tissues and organs in the laboratory and safely implanting them when the body cannot heal itself.

Developments in DNA repair, stem cell therapy and cloning will empower such advances to become a reality in the very near future. Importantly, regenerative medicine has the potential to solve the problem of the shortage of organs available for donation compared to the number of patients requiring life-saving organ transplants, as well as bypassing organ transplant rejection issues, since the new organs cells will have been grown to order and perfectly match those of the patient.

A good example comes from the field of Dentistry. Many of us have had problems with our teeth over the years, not only is it hard to find a good Dentist and get an appointment, but the costs can be astronomical when paying out of pocket. Developing the concept of the self-repairing tooth is something that researchers at the Leeds Dental Institute have been working on for several years. Professor Jennifer Kirkham's team have recently developed a peptide-based paste which coats the surface of teeth. This forms a gel in the pores of the enamel (which may be chronically damaged), creating a scaffold that attracts minerals such as calcium, and helps to regenerate the surface structure of the tooth [2]. This pain-free, non-surgical option for repairing corrupted teeth has shown very promising results and if it can be replicated in larger trials they are expecting the treatment to be available in dental practices in 2–3 years' time. Eventually one might expect to see this technology into the toothpastes that we use every day and have a cumulatively positive and protective effect. Anything that reduces visits to the Dentist sounds like an important advance.

Think then, of regenerative medicine as a way of restoring function by taking advantage of molecular and cellular mechanisms at a very foundational level and using the biological machinery of cells to fix, renew or grow a new body system, set of tissues or entire organ.

Where Do Stem Cells Come From?

These are one of the key components of regenerative medicine. Stem cells (often referred to as progenitors) can differentiate into various different cell types, to repair damaged tissues. They are the body's raw material, the building blocks from which all other cell types are derived. Nerve cells, blood cells, muscle cells, heart cells and gut cells all start off as lowly stem cells. During embryonic development the stem cells divide and replicate to form offspring called daughter cells. It's these daughter cells which then change into new forms with specialised functions. No other cell type is able to create other cell types hence the interest in their powerful abilities.

Stem cells can be derived from human embryos that are a few days old. This small collection of cells contains 'pluri-potent' stem cells which can differentiate into either more stem cells or any type of human body cell. This versatility has triggered great scientific interest and potential but is not without controversy given the nature of the material and the attitude of various groups towards the use of embryos as a source of therapy.

Perinatal stem cells can be harvested from both amniotic fluid and cord blood, and these have the ability to change into specialised cells. Forward thinking bio-tech companies have already cottoned on to the possible commercial aspects of encouraging new parents to save some cord blood when their baby is born, and they can bank the samples for future need.

Humans continue to have stem cells throughout their life and are found in small volumes in most adult tissues such as in the bone marrow or in fat cells. They can give rise to new cell types but are much more limited than embryonic or perinatal stem cells. New research evidence suggests that under the right circumstances adult stem cells can be provoked into changing into different cell types such as cardiac muscle cells, and testing is ongoing.

Stem cells can be guided (via genetic programming) into becoming new and different cell types with specific purposes and at the same time avoid immune rejection by host defence systems. This therefore provides the possibility of generating new cells to fix damaged or lost tissues such as pancreatic islet cells (to make some insulin) in the context of Diabetes where the original cells have been destroyed, or to grow new nerve cells in a person with a neurological condition like Parkinson's disease.

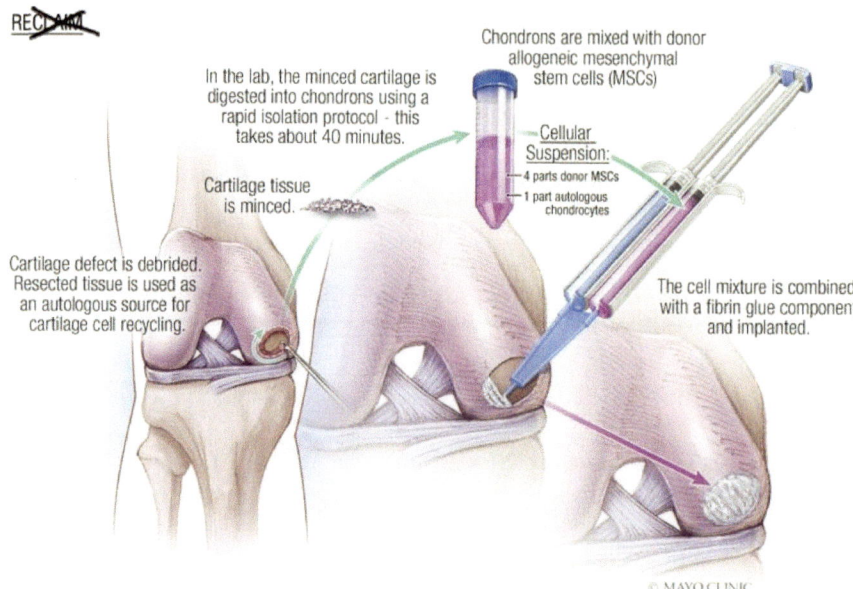

Fig. 9.2 Overview of knee cartilage stem cell repair. Image Source: Reproduced with permission of Mayo Foundation for Medical Education and Research, all rights reserved (https://www.mayo-clinic.org/medical-professionals/orthopedic-surgery/news/novel-stem-cell-therapy-for-repair-of-knee-cartilage/mac-20450891)

Stem cell-based therapies have shown promise in restoring vision in animal models with retinal degeneration, offering hope for treating blindness and vision-related disorders. Similarly, there is a role in corneal regeneration, stem cell therapy has shown promise in regenerating corneal tissue for vision restoration. Other applications include bone marrow repair—haematopoietic stem cell transplants are used to treat blood-related disorders like leukaemia and lymphoma. There is also a great deal of research exploring the use of stem cells to repair damaged heart muscle tissue after heart attacks and other cardiac conditions. Additionally, the wear and tear damage found in osteoarthritis is seen as an important target for regenerative repair of damaged cartilage, given the pain and restriction in mobility this condition causes for so many people (see Fig. 9.2 below).

Tissue Engineering Regenerative medicine also involves creating functional tissues and organs in the laboratory by growing sheets of new cells under optimum conditions. This can lead to advancements like; artificial skin—lab-grown skin can be used for burn victims and in cosmetic testing or bioengineered bladders grown from a patient's own cells which have already been transplanted successfully. One of the big success stories to hit the news in recent years was the creation of an entirely new trachea, grown on a scaffold, that was successfully transplanted into a 30 year old Colombian woman with a damaged airway, by a team led by Professor Paolo Macchiarini, in Barcelona in 2008 and which didn't require immunosuppression [3].

Gene Therapy Gene therapy is a method which alters an individual's genetic information to treat or cure illnesses. This can take place through the replacement of a defective gene with a healthy copy. This switches off the disease causing gene and introduces a new or modified gene to help overcome the effects of disease. Gene therapy plays a role in regenerating tissues by correcting genetic defects—fixing faulty code. In conditions such as Spinal Muscular Atrophy (SMA) gene therapies have been developed to treat this disorder which affects motor neuron functioning. The CRISPR-Cas9 gene-editing technology has enabled precise modification of genes, which can be applied in regenerative medicine to correct genetic defects, create personalised therapies, and enhance the safety and efficacy of regenerative treatments.

mRNA Vaccines Although primarily associated with vaccination, mRNA technology has the potential to be used in regenerative medicine to stimulate tissue regeneration. This technology was demonstrated in the context of heart regeneration in animal studies. If modified mRNA is delivered after an experimental heart attack, the signalling mechanism that it induces transiently allows cardiac cells to proliferate, leading to a reduction in volume of the damaged cardiac area and subsequent improvement in heart performance [4].

Organ Transplantation Whilst the ultimate goal is to build an entirely new organ for transplanting into a human with a faulty organ, regenerative medicine techniques are already improving the outcomes of existing organ transplants procedures. In diabetes treatment, pancreatic islet cell transplantation can restore insulin production in some patients. In Cardiology, scientists are working on growing heart tissues for transplantation and drug testing. In the speciality of Hepatology, researchers have made progress in growing functional human liver tissue in the laboratory, which could have implications for liver transplantation and drug testing (and implications for our societal thoughts about the commonest cause of liver failure—alcohol).

3D Bioprinting Advancements in 3D bioprinting technology have allowed for the creation of complex tissue structures, including vascular networks and scaffolds, which are crucial for the successful transplantation of lab-grown organs.

Wound Healing Regenerative approaches can significantly improve wound healing, especially in chronic wounds; Platelet-Rich Plasma (PRP) therapy uses a patient's own blood components to stimulate tissue repair and can accelerate wound healing. PRP is commonly used by athletes to promote healing of injuries like tendonitis.

Neurological Disorders Research is exploring ways to repair and regenerate damaged nervous tissue, which is notoriously slow and hard to grow for repair purposes. Neural stem cells are being investigated for conditions like spinal cord injuries and neurodegenerative diseases. Research in neural regeneration has made progress in addressing brain and spinal cord injuries, including the use of stem cells and bioengineered scaffolds.

Dermal Fillers In the field of aesthetic medicine dermal fillers contain substances that stimulate collagen production, enhancing skin elasticity which will be relevant in the multi-billion-dollar cosmetic market.

Vascular Regeneration Cardiovascular disease is the biggest killer in the western world and is caused by atherosclerotic damage to the inner lining of the blood vessels that supply critical parts of the human body. Regenerative approaches are being explored to treat vascular diseases to help improve cardiovascular health. Researchers at Cytograft Tissue Engineering in the US have developed a technique in which epithelial skin cells are removed from a patient's hand [5]. These cell types produce large amounts of the connective tissue collagen which is strong and elastic. This harvest is then grown in laboratory conditions and infused with nutrients to form a thin sheet of tissue which can then be rolled into hollow tube structures. This is then lined with another cell type taken from the internal surface of superficial veins. Blood vessels up to 20 cm in length have been manufactured using a combination of patients own cells and donor cells to create a transplant ready blood vessel. These new veins can then be used for a variety of 'plumbing' related needs, such as creating better fistula sites for patients receiving kidney dialysis. Cytograft's founder Nicolas L'Heureux describes how they are using a completely human fibre from which they can now build all kinds of structures by weaving, braiding, knitting or a combination of techniques [6].

CAR-T Cell Therapies A major challenge in introducing many of these regenerative techniques originates from the body's understandable desire to attack foreign agents, this limits many of the approaches to bodily repair that have been tried in the past. Patients fortunate enough to receive organ transplants must take combinations of anti-rejection therapies which themselves have a number of significant side effects such as susceptibility to infections. T-Cells are types of white blood cell (lymphocytes) and a big player in the immune rejection response. By removing T-cells from the body, genetically modifying them and then re-infusing them into an individual, scientists have found a way to dampen down a patient's aggressive immune reaction. CAR stands for chimeric antigen receptor. CAR-T cells are designed to recognise and target a specific protein on cancer cells such as in the context of leukaemia. While primarily used in cancer treatment, CAR-T cell therapies demonstrate the potential to target and eliminate harmful immune responses, making them relevant in autoimmune conditions and regenerative medicine.

Exosome-Based Therapies Exosomes are small vesicles secreted by cells, they have gained attention for their role in cell-to-cell communication and regenerative potential. Exosome-based therapies are being explored for tissue repair and regeneration. They are thought to have immunomodulatory effects and are being studied as a potential treatment for inflammatory and autoimmune disorders such as rheumatoid arthritis and multiple sclerosis [7].

These approaches and examples demonstrate the diverse applications of regenerative medicine, ranging from life-saving treatments for serious diseases to cosmetic enhancements. As research continues, regenerative medicine holds great promise for improving the quality of life for many individuals and addressing a wide range of medical conditions. Such breakthroughs offer hope for the development of innovative treatments for a wide range of diseases and conditions, ultimately improving the quality of life for patients—but also having a significant impact on how care will be delivered in the future.

Changing Hospitals

Health services will need to transform to accommodate the changes that regenerative medicine will bring. Technology plays a significant part in this, not just in the development of regenerative medicine advances themselves, but also in terms of the surveillance and capture systems around how and when to utilise such advances. When I first became a Consultant, I rewarded myself with the purchase of a shiny, second hand (probably third hand) BMW Coupe. Taking it to the official dealership for servicing (not some random garage) was very satisfying, especially for the customer service, and I was intrigued how at check in, the assistant would take my key fob, place it on the special reader, which downloaded all of my car's latest data, and be able to inform me that my rear brake pads would need replacing in 2000 miles time. They knew the status of all the car's internal systems, the oil level was running a little low so they could top that up for me, but also my gearbox was becoming problematic and on its way out. I'd need a new one, expensive, but they could order it for me and have it installed in a couple of days' time. Such diagnostic speed and prognostic accuracy amazed and delighted me. This ability to know what needed to be fixed, what needed to be replaced, and when, felt remarkable back in the early 2010s. How fantastic would it be to transfer such capabilities to the medical realm.

It is thought that the term *regenerative medicine* first came from an article by Leland Kaiser on Hospital Administration published in 1992 [8]. The end of the article outlines several new technologies that are likely to have an impact on the work of Hospitals in the future. He outlines how 'Regenerative Medicine' is 'a new branch of medicine that attempts to change the course of chronic disease and in many instances will regenerate tired and failing organ systems'. Indeed, over 30 years on we can contemplate that it will shift the work of Hospitals in two main ways. Firstly, a move towards more MOT-like surveillance, monitoring and tracking of physiological markers and organ functions over time—perhaps through a combination of remote monitors, internal body sensors and automated diagnostics (remember the smart toilet) linked through the cloud—being able to predict or calculate signs of deterioration and activate treatment or avoidance measures. And secondly, as a spare parts replacement service, generating new organs to order, which can then be inserted, connected or plumbed in at a time of your convenience (and when the robot surgeon is available). All of this of course will avoid the old-fashioned notion of rejection and the need for toxic immuno-suppressant drugs, because the new tissues and organs will be grown and tailored to be immuno-typed to the individual. Could Hospitals undergo a major transition in which they purely deal with either acute emergencies or trauma and nothing else because all other problems are solved by the spare parts industry which has eliminated the vast bulk of human disease?

The Implications of Regenerative Medicine

This may all seem rather fanciful but remember that we used to live in a world in which people died from a simple scratch and computers would fill warehouses. As technologies develop, the ways in which we live our lives and that we practice medicine will change profoundly and have many positive impacts on healthcare delivery.

Tissue Repair and Replacement Regenerative medicine can repair or replace damaged or diseased tissues and organs, offering new hope to patients with conditions that were previously considered untreatable or required organ transplantation. Similarly in the context of trauma and injuries regenerative therapies can improve outcomes for conditions such as spinal cord injuries, by promoting tissue repair and regeneration, potentially enabling patients to regain lost function. Alongside this, there will be improved healing and recovery, regenerative therapies can accelerate the healing process for various injuries, surgeries, and chronic wounds, reducing pain and recovery times.

Reduced Reliance on Organ Donors Regenerative approaches can decrease the demand for organ donors and the risk of organ rejection, as tissues and organs can be engineered from a patient's own cells. If it is possible to utilise laboratory grown organs and tissues, then the demand and competition for donor organs will drop dramatically and also remove the need for organ recipients to have to take lifelong toxic medications to control the risk of immune rejection.

Personalised Medicine Treatments will be increasingly tailored to an individual's unique genetic makeup, reducing the risk of adverse reactions and optimising treatment effectiveness. Using a patient's own cells and modifying the genetic code of immune components or foreign tissues can help to make treatments more effective and eliminate side-effects. For example, there is hope that this approach can enhance cancer treatments by improving targeted therapies and minimising damage to healthy tissues.

Treatment of Previously Incurable Diseases Conditions which currently have limited or no treatment options, such as neurodegenerative diseases and certain genetic disorders, may benefit from regenerative approaches. This offers promise to patients and their families where there was previously no hope of any treatment.

Treatment of Age-Related Conditions Modern medicine has helped people live longer but their 'health span', the amount of time spent in good health can still be diminished. Regenerative medicine may offer solutions for age-related conditions, such as osteoarthritis and age-related macular degeneration, potentially improving the quality of life for elderly individuals, as well as the duration. By addressing age-related diseases and promoting tissue repair, it will allow people to enjoy more active and fulfilling lives as they age.

Enhanced Quality of Life Regenerative therapies can restore lost or impaired functions, improving the quality of life for individuals with disabilities or chronic illnesses.

Long-Term Cost Savings and Reduced Healthcare Burden While the initial costs of regenerative therapies can be high, they may lead to long-term cost savings by reducing the need for continuous treatments, hospitalisations, and ongoing medical care. By preventing or curing diseases altogether, regenerative medicine can alleviate the burden on healthcare systems and improve the overall health of populations. This will help to reduce capacity constraints. In cases where organ transplantation is necessary, regenerative medicine can help reduce waiting times and the associated risks for patients in need.

Economic Benefits Medical technology can stimulate economic growth through research and development, healthcare services, and the creation of jobs in biotechnology and healthcare industries. It already fosters international collaboration among researchers, institutions, and healthcare providers, leading to the sharing of knowledge and the acceleration of scientific advancements. It will also mean healthy workers returning to the workforce and reduce the numbers of people dependent on health and disability payouts.

Overall, regenerative medicine holds tremendous promise for society, transforming healthcare by providing new treatment options, improving patient outcomes, and offering solutions for a wide range of medical conditions. As research and technology in this field continue to advance, the positive implications are likely to become even more pronounced, benefiting individuals and societies alike.

The Downsides of Disruption Through Regenerative Medicine

Regenerative medicine is a promising field with the potential to revolutionise healthcare, but it also faces several significant challenges and obstacles that need to be addressed for its successful development and widespread application. There are a large and interesting range of ethical, regulatory, and accessibility challenges that need to be carefully addressed to ensure equitable and responsible use.

Ethical and Moral Concerns The use of certain regenerative techniques for research and treatment, such as embryonic stem cells, raises ethical and moral dilemmas, as it involves the destruction of human embryos. This issue has led to debates about when life begins and the moral status of embryos. These concerns can lead to regulatory restrictions, public debates, campaigns, misinformation and misunderstanding.

Ownership and Control of Genetic Material The use of genetic material, including gene editing technologies, raises concerns about ownership and control of genetic information and the potential for misuse. The well documented case of Henrietta Lacks whose cancer cells are the origins of the *HeLa* immortalised cell line demonstrates how tissues might be taken without consent and used for a whole range of research and commercial purposes further down the line [9]. This is a warning from history about privacy and patient rights.

The case of Dr. He Jiankui, an associate Professor from Shenzhen, provides a salient lesson in bioethical controversy. This Chinese fertility scientist changed the genetic code of human embryos in 2018, to remove the risk of them developing infection with the HIV virus, (by removing the CCR5 gene) and these were subsequently implanted via IVF, and gave rise to the world's first genetically edited babies—twin girls called Lulu and Nana. At first this was described as a historical breakthrough in the application of gene editing technology for disease prevention [10]. However, when more details came out this intervention received widespread condemnation because of his unlawful research, and he was found guilty by the Chinese authorities of forging documents and unethical conduct. Following this Dr. He and his colleagues were fined and imprisoned as well as being banned from working in fertility medicine for life.

In 2019, the Chinese Academy of Medical Sciences announced, *"We are opposed to any clinical operation of human embryo genome editing for reproductive purposes in violation of laws, regulations, and ethical norms in the absence of full scientific evaluation. In the rapidly developing area of genome editing technology, our scientific community should uphold the highest standards of bioethics in undertaking responsible biomedical research and applications"* [11].

Safety and Efficacy Ensuring the safety and efficacy of regenerative therapies is a major challenge. The unknown long-term effects of regenerative therapies can pose ethical dilemmas. Patients and researchers may not have a complete understanding of potential risks, including the problems of immune rejection, development of cancer, or unintended consequences. Researchers must demonstrate that these treatments not only work but also have acceptable risks and side effects. Long-term safety data is so far lacking given the early stages of development and limited roll out of new technologies. Randomised controlled trials will be needed to provide assurance. The long-term effects and outcomes of regenerative therapies are not always well understood, and long-term follow-up studies are needed to assess their safety and durability.

Informed Consent Ensuring that patients fully understand the experimental and sometimes risky nature of regenerative treatments is essential. Obtaining informed consent can be tricky, particularly when patients may be desperate for potential cures. Balancing the respect for patient autonomy with the potential for unproven and risky regenerative treatments can be ethically challenging. Patients have the right to make decisions about their own care, but this must be done with a clear understanding of the risks and benefits.

Tumour Formation Some stem cell-based therapies carry a risk of forming tumours or promoting uncontrolled cell growth, particularly if the cells used are not fully differentiated or controlled properly, they have the potential to proliferate and grow into anything. Uncontrolled, unregulated cell growth is also known as metaplasia or neoplasia (which are synonyms for pre-cancer and cancer).

Regulatory Hurdles Regenerative medicine faces complex and evolving regulatory frameworks. Striking the right balance between fostering innovation and ensuring patient safety will be a continual challenge, especially in the face of political and religious groups with their own agendas and misunderstandings. Collaboration among researchers and institutions worldwide is essential, but regulatory differences across countries can hinder progress and restrict global access to treatments.

Access and Equity There is a concern that regenerative medicine treatments may only be available to those who can afford them, leading to issues of healthcare inequality. Ensuring equitable access to these therapies is an ethical imperative. The proliferation of unproven or fraudulent regenerative treatments, often offered by private clinics outside of regulatory oversight, can lead to ethical concerns regarding patient safety, false hope, and exploitation.

High Costs Developing and implementing regenerative therapies will be expensive, making them inaccessible to many. Reducing costs while maintaining quality is essential for wider adoption and may take a long time to achieve like with many new technologies. Developing personalised regenerative therapies for each patient will be time-consuming and expensive. Streamlining the process and making it more cost-effective is going to be a challenge. Scaling up the production of regenerative products to meet the demand of a larger population can be a logistical and technical problem. However, in time we may all have our own home stem cell repair kit tucked away in the bathroom cabinet above the smart toilet.

Standardisation and Quality Control Ensuring consistency in the manufacturing and quality of regenerative products can be challenging. Standardisation and rigorous quality control processes will be vital. The ethical (and legal) obligation to provide consistent and high-quality care means that regenerative therapies must meet rigorous standards and quality control measures. Failure to do so can harm patients and erode trust in the field.

Intellectual Property and Commercialisation Disputes over intellectual property rights and commercial interests can delay the development and roll out of regenerative therapies. Ethical concerns can arise when commercial interests prioritise profit over patient well-being. Conflicts of interest may affect research and decision-making regarding the development and promotion of regenerative therapies.

Clinical Trial Design Designing clinical trials for regenerative therapies will be complex due to the unique nature of these treatments. Finding appropriate control groups and endpoints is going to be difficult. Ethical concerns include the need for transparency in research, clinical trials, and the reporting of results to avoid conflicts of interest and ensure that data is not selectively presented.

Risk of Enhancement and Non-Therapeutic Use Regenerative technologies may be used for non-therapeutic purposes, such as enhancing physical or cognitive capabilities, raising ethical questions about the boundaries of medical intervention. We've already seen in the fields of athletics and cosmetics the extent that people will go to enhance normal human physiology and attributes for a competitive advantage.

Addressing these challenges requires collaboration among researchers, healthcare providers, regulatory bodies, industry stakeholders, policy makers, ethicists, clinicians and patient groups. Continued research, investment, and innovation are essential to overcome these obstacles and unlock the full potential of regenerative medicine for improving healthcare outcomes and patient quality of life.

The Medical Consultation of the Near Future

The clinic room door swishes open and Mrs. Carter strides in.

"Welcome back Mrs. Carter, you're looking better than ever, come and take a seat. It's time for your annual review".

"Hello Doctor, nice to see you, where are you today?"

"In Barbados again for the cricket, weather's terrible though" he announces from the video screen. "Let's get your details then".

"Do you want me to scan my thumb print Doctor?" asks Mrs. Carter.

"No need, the clinic room chair has just measured all of your physiological information and I've got the downloads from your home monitoring system".

"Is everything alright?" she asks tentatively, "I haven't had any alerts recently".

"Blood pressure's up a bit today, but that's probably the excitement of coming to the clinic!"

"Yes, I've not had a high blood pressure reading for a long time now Doctor, ever since you got me that new kidney. It was lovely to come off of all that medication after so long".

"Good to hear that. Are you on any medication at all now?"

"No, nothing really, just some bone supplements to stop my arthritis coming back. I had the stem cells but I used to have awful back and knee pains so don't want that to come back".

"Fine fine, and do you do anything for stress now as I see on your notes that that used to be a problem" he asks.

"Well I have taken up smoking again. It really helps calm me down Doctor, but I only have five a day at the moment".

"Ok that's fine, you could always increase and go up to 10 or 20 a day if you need to. I remember when I was a medical student people used to say that smoking was bad for you, but that was before artificial lungs, so smoke away that's what I say".

"Thank you, Doctor, that's very kind. So do my tests and readings indicate that I need to do anything different then".

"No, it looks like everything is ticking along very nicely Mrs. Carter. The genetic readouts are excellent. All of your components are running well and are still under guarantee. You carry on doing what you're doing, and the remote monitoring will let us know if anything goes wrong well in advance. I think that it's all going very well".

"Oh that's lovely to hear. Not bad for 108 years old Doctor. Goodbye".

References

1. Chagastelles PC, Nardi NB. Biology of stem cells: an overview. Kidney Int Suppl. 2011;1(3):63–7. https://doi.org/10.1038/kisup.2011.15.
2. Kirkham J, Firth A, Vernals D, et al. Self-assembling peptide scaffolds promote enamel remineralization. J Dent Res. 2007;86(5):426–30. https://doi.org/10.1177/154405910708600507.
3. Wise J. Five year results show success of first tissue engineered trachea transplant. BMJ. 2013;347:f6365. https://doi.org/10.1136/bmj.f6365.
4. Zangi L, Lui KO, von Gise A, et al. Modified mRNA directs the fate of heart progenitor cells and induces vascular regeneration after myocardial infarction. Nat Biotechnol. 2013;31(10):898–907.
5. L'Heureux N, McAllister T. Cytograft tissue engineering: a new paradigm in cardiovascular tissue engineering. Regen Med. 2008;3:471–5. https://doi.org/10.2217/17460751.3.4.471.
6. Federation of American Societies for Experimental Biology (FASEB). Making human textiles: research team ups the ante with development of blood vessels woven from donor cells. ScienceDaily. 2012 Apr 23. www.sciencedaily.com/releases/2012/04/120423131512.htm. Accessed 18 Jun 2024.
7. Muthu S, Bapat A, Jain R, Jeyaraman N, Jeyaraman M. Exosomal therapy-a new frontier in regenerative medicine. Stem Cell Investig. 2021;8:7. https://doi.org/10.21037/sci-2020-037.
8. Kaiser LR. The future of multihospital systems. Top Health Care Financ. 1992 Summer;18(4):32–45.

9. Skloot R. The immortal life of Henrietta Lacks. London: Picador; 2018.
10. Li JR, Walker S, Nie JB, Zhang XQ. Experiments that led to the first gene-edited babies: the ethical failings and the urgent need for better governance. J Zhejiang Univ Sci B. 2019;20(1):32–8. https://doi.org/10.1631/jzus.B1800624.
11. Wang C, Zhai X, Zhang X, Li L, Wang J, Liu DP. Gene-edited babies: Chinese Academy of Medical Sciences' response and action. Lancet. 2019;393(10166):25–6. https://doi.org/10.1016/S0140-6736(18)33080-0.

Further Reading

Petrigliano FA, Liu NQ, Lee S, et al. Long-term repair of porcine articular cartilage using cryopreservable, clinically compatible human embryonic stem cell-derived chondrocytes. NPJ Regen Med. 2021;6:77. https://doi.org/10.1038/s41536-021-00187-3.

Chapter 10
The Smart Hospital

Abstract A 'smart hospital' is a healthcare institution that uses advanced technologies and integrated systems to enhance patient care, improve operational efficiency and streamline healthcare processes. The concept of smart hospitals represents a paradigm shift in healthcare delivery, driven by the integration of advanced technologies, such as Internet of Things (IoT) devices, artificial intelligence (AI), big data analytics, data-driven solutions, and more patient-centric care. We explore how these technologies could enhance patient care delivery, smooth operations, and promote data fuelled decision-making around many aspects of healthcare.

This chapter also highlights the challenges that smart hospitals face, including the high implementation costs, interoperability issues, and the staff training and capability requirements. It emphasises the importance of regulatory compliance and the need for scalability to accommodate future growth. We underscore the transformative potential of smart hospitals in improving health outcomes, patient engagement, and addressing the evolving healthcare landscape. It explores real-world examples of successful smart hospital implementations and offers insights into the path forwards as healthcare institutions worldwide embark on the journey toward smarter, more efficient, and user-friendly care delivery.

Keywords Smart hospital · Digital hospital · Intelligent hospital · Remote monitoring · Fabric technology · Electronic medical records · Digitisation · EMRAM · HIMSS · Smart hospital standards

What Is a Smart Hospital?

In response to increased health demands and expectations, it remains a fundamental approach of governments and health systems to want to build new physical Hospitals. Massive construction projects around the globe, especially in the developing world, for example in India, have seen significant numbers of modern Hospitals being built at vast expense. Indeed, in the UK, the NHS is investing in '40' new hospitals as part of the adventurous new hospitals programme (NHP). This is despite the fact that we know an increasing amount of medical work, diagnostics, management and care can be delivered outside of the traditional bricks and mortar setting. There will of course always be the requirement for a focused clinical location in which to look after those with the greatest care needs, but modern healthcare planning is slow to consider the future of medicine including virtual models of care—this may be because if you disaggregate the patient from a physical care setting, you lose the sense of ownership and responsibility, or is it because we're not yet ready to let go of the concept of our shiny, white, medical palaces as a focal point for centralised healthcare?

We have so far shown that it is possible to have the concept of clinics, wards and hospitals without walls and deliver medical care in new and interesting ways (emergency care, primary care, out-patient care and even some aspects of in-patient care can be provided remotely, safely and cost effectively). For those that do need to remain in Hospital beds there is an exciting selection of digital solutions that seek to enhance the way that Hospitals function, bringing them to new levels of efficiency and productivity. This chapter looks at the principle of the 'smart hospital' and examines how it can align with virtual hospital models of care.

The 'digitally enabled hospital' is a concept that emerged in the early 2000's in Korea, with the goal of fostering a complete transformation from analogue hospital workflows where medication charts, X-ray films, order slips, paper medical records and pens were mostly used for all aspects of recording patients' medical histories, to a digital hospital workflow involving the "four 'lesses'" (filmless, chartless, slipless, paperless) method, by establishing computerised physician order-entry, picture archiving and communication systems (PACS), electronic medical record (EMR) systems, and hospital administrative/business systems.

A smart hospital, takes things a step further and can be described as a healthcare institution that utilises advanced technologies, data-driven strategies, and integrated systems to enhance patient care, improve operational efficiency, and optimise the overall healthcare experience for both patients and providers by being fully interconnected and responsive. The Seoul Asan Hospital Innovation Design Centre have defined this as;

> A next-generation hospital that exceeds the limits of existing hospitals in terms of quality of care, patient safety, patient experience, and productivity by using technologies related to the fourth industrial revolution [1].

The concept of a smart hospital therefore revolves around leveraging advanced technologies, digital health interventions and data to create a healthcare facility that is highly efficient, patient-centred, and capable of delivering high-quality care. Smart hospital services can be classified into the following types: services based on location recognition and tracking technology that measures and monitors the location information of an object based on short-range communication technology such as Bluetooth or ZigBee (providing you with real time bed status and porter location for example); high-speed communication network-based services based on new wireless communication technology; Internet of Things-based services that connect objects embedded with sensors and communication functions to the internet; mobile health services such as mobile phones, tablets, and wearables (smart devices);

Table 10.1 Summary table of smart hospital components

Core element	Description
Digitisation of all information	All information generated in hospitals needs to be available and accessible (along role-based lines) and stored in a separate and structured format for use in reporting and analysis whenever possible, aiming for an automated, paperless workflow.
Provision of stable core infrastructure	Stable high-speed networking, perfect identification technology, and interconnection of sensor networks and embedded systems.
Integration of technologies	A wide range of technologies, including the Internet of Things (IoT) sensors, artificial intelligence (AI), big data analytics, machine learning, and automation, to improve various aspects of healthcare delivery. The most important aspect is that such systems are interoperable and can communicate effectively with one another. There should be minimal use of proprietary systems and the benefit of successful integration is that you can develop a better approach to operational delivery through either an intelligent building management system or a clinical command centre. Hitachi, for example have rolled out a networked clinical command system in the Royal Salford Hospital in the UK, which because of the successful data integration and insights, allowed average length of Hospital stay to come down by 3 days within 3 weeks of going live.
Mobile integrated systems	All resources, such as people, equipment, and technology, should be supported to be as mobile as possible to support flexibility and decision making at the point of care.
Establishment of a unified communication system	Communication and collaboration systems work through the integration of audio, video and data, allowing smooth and safe communication between all stakeholders (patients, clinicians, managers and administrators).
System automation	All of the above should be able to contribute to an improved patient treatment experience by increasing the efficiency and productivity of hospital operations through automation wherever possible.
Data analytics and predictive tools	Smart hospitals harness the power of data analytics to make informed decisions. They use predictive analytics to identify trends, disease outbreaks, and potential patient issues (such as physiological deterioration) before they become critical.

AI-based services for the diagnosis and prediction of diseases; robot services provided on behalf of humans in various medical fields (from portering, to pharmacy organisation to surgery); extended reality services that apply hyper-realistic immersive technology to medical practice; and telehealth using IT services [2]. The key elements that define a smart hospital are outlined below (Table 10.1).

The primary focus of a smart hospital should be on providing patient-centred care. This means tailoring healthcare services to meet the individual needs, preferences, and expectations of patients, while also involving patients in decision-making about their care. Smart hospitals promote patient activation and engagement through mobile apps, patient portals, and educational resources. Patients are empowered with information to actively participate in their healthcare journey (if they want to be). The concept of a smart hospital therefore reflects a commitment to continuously improving the quality of care, enhancing operational efficiency, and embracing innovation to meet the evolving healthcare needs of patients and communities. While technology plays a central role as an enabler, the ultimate goal is to provide compassionate, safe, and effective healthcare services.

Global Exemplars

The business case for smart hospitals is already very strong. In most OECD countries, implementing digital solutions in hospitals and healthcare delivery could help realise cost savings of more than 10% of overall national healthcare expenditure. Business investors have recognised the opportunity—venture capital funding for digital health solutions has increased exponentially, from about US $1 billion in 2011 to more than US $8 billion in 2018 [2]. New Hospitals are being built and old ones replaced around the world all the time. If you construct a new Hospital in the present you must bear in mind the future models of healthcare delivery, especially given the long lead times with regards to planning, design, consultation and construction. A Hospital that is due to open in 2035 is going to look, feel and behave very differently to a present-day Hospital. There are multiple examples of good practice from around the world that have already absorbed this challenge.

Dublin Children's Hospital Under construction at the time of writing, this new children's healthcare facility seeks to be a world class site, with 380 individual en-suite in-patient bedrooms, co-located with a children's health research and innovation centre (Fig. 10.1).

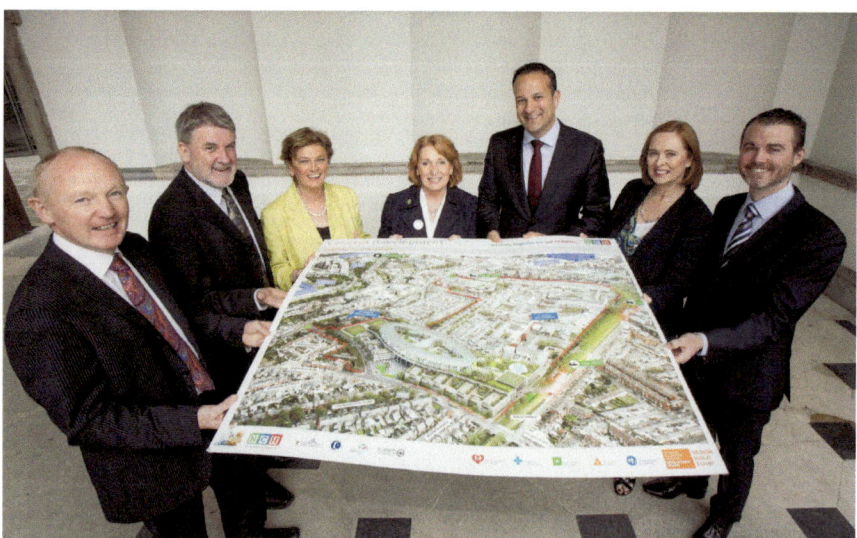

Fig. 10.1 The launch of plans for the new Dublin Children's hospital. Image Credit: Naoise Culhane (https://www.flickr.com/photos/doh-ireland/18963302098) Reproduced under Creative Commons Licence BY 2.0 Deed. https://creativecommons.org/licenses/by/2.0/

When it opens it will be the first public hospital in Ireland which has had a significant investment in ICT data infrastructure. With healthcare innovation evolving at a rapid rate, the Health Executive understands that future-proofing the hospital is key to facilitating the optimal delivery of current and developing clinical best practice. Eilísh Hardiman, Chief Executive of Children's Health Ireland said *"We're going to be what we call 'born digital'. It's easier to be born digital than trying to make some of the changes that are happening within the existing system"* [3]. The new children's Hospital will incorporate technologies such as a clinical command centre to provide an overview of patient status and operational flow, as well as automated guided vehicles (AGV's) to transport equipment, laundry and waste around the site in order to improve service and efficiency and sophisticated systems such as intelligent building management (or Digital Twin) which can monitor and diagnose problems within the fabric of the Hospital and prioritise repair and maintenance.

Cleveland Clinical Abu Dhabi (United Arab Emirates) This is a multispecialty hospital known for its advanced use of technology (Fig. 10.2). The hospital incorporates smart systems for patient care, including robotics for surgeries, telemedicine, and an integrated electronic health record (EHR) system. Examples include Transpara an imaging system that is already equipped with artificial intelligence which supports breast cancer screening, and an in-house automated medication dispensing system—this streamlines workflow and reduces the types of medication errors that come from using handwritten paper prescriptions. Everything is connected to the right patient through the use of a barcode ID on the patient's wristband making sure that the correct drug is given to the right patient at the right time and any allergy information is automatically flagged. It is ranked as one of the top smart Hospitals in the world by a number of authorities [4].

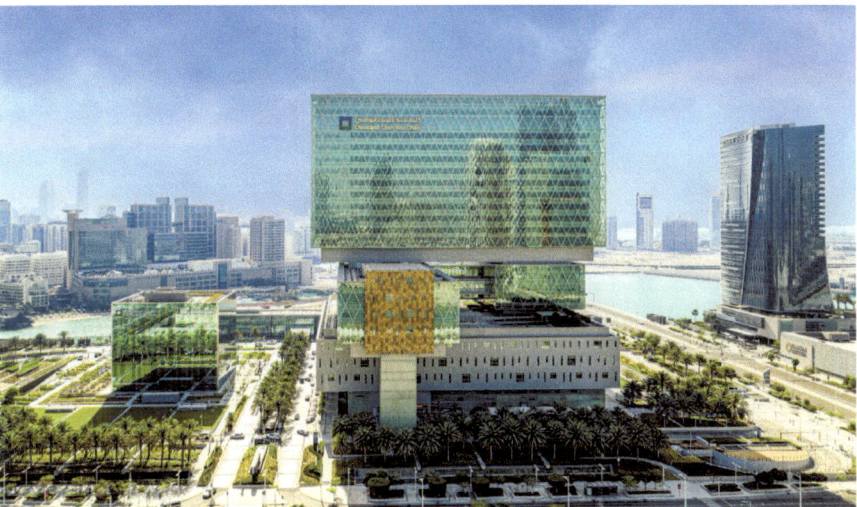

Fig. 10.2 The Cleveland Clinic, Abu Dhabi. Source: Cleveland Clinic—reproduced with kind permission (unmodified)

Karolinska University Hospital This is one of Europe's leading Hospitals and has been on a journey to incorporate the latest and most useful digital solutions in order to enhance patient care delivery (Fig. 10.3). Alongside this the Hospital has taken the opportunity to take a transformative step in how care is provided. The traditional approach to having distinct clinical departments has been abolished and healthcare delivery at the Karolinska has been focussed on the patient journey and the flow of their care. The new operating model strengthens cooperation between different disciplines by integrating care delivery from specialists in emergency care, surgery, medical teams, and imaging experts for example, by placing them in the same building or corridor, with the aim of combining their skills and experience to work more effectively for the patient at the centre, rather than their own domains. Patrick Puhony, the operational director of imaging has said *"We are transforming from a central radiology department into a function that is spread out across multiple buildings. We want to be in close vicinity to our patients and to referring clinicians, so that we can deliver the best value to them. We do not simply want to provide a CT scan. We want to provide an answer to a medical question"* [5]. This is an admirable aim and eliminates one of the barriers in medical care delivery, something that is difficult to achieve without a commitment to organisational development and change management—something that is often very challenging in a healthcare environment.

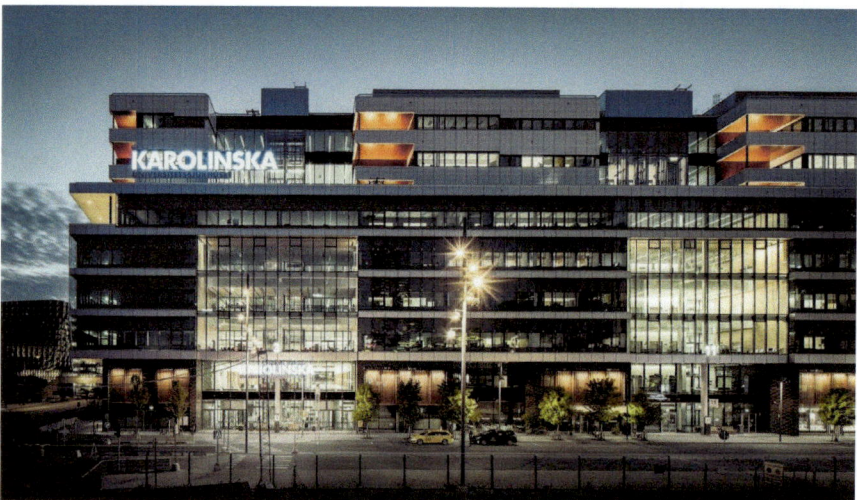

Fig. 10.3 The new Karolinska Institute Hospital. Credit: Felix Gerlach and Tengbom Architects. Kindly reproduced with permission

What Types of Technologies Do You Find in a Smart Hospital?

The approach to designing a smart Hospital starts well in advance of the physical build programme. There needs to be a consideration of the foundational infrastructure technologies that a modern smart building requires, so that these can be planned and considered early. Hospitals are increasingly technology dependent so high-speed internet cabling and internal mobile data networks for example need to be embedded in the fabric of the building, as so many other technologies are reliant on them to be present with good coverage and bandwidth to cope with high demands. Medical and building technology is also becoming increasingly dependent on sensor networks to pick up and process information remotely and convey it back to a centralised system, be it a clinical command centre to track patient vital signs, or a digital twin that monitors the health of the building. On top of this you then need to think about all of the clinical and management systems that allow you to operate a modern Hospital effectively—such as electronic medication prescribing and administration. The HIMSS (Healthcare Information and Management Systems Society) model is currently the standard being used to assess the digital maturity of a healthcare facility and one can only achieve the highest levels (each eight-stage (0–7) maturity model operates as a vendor-neutral roadmap for success and offers global benchmarking) if you have fully integrated systems and have made the leap to being paper free. The table below (Table 10.2) demonstrates how the scoring system works in relation to electronic medical records adoption (known as EMRAM) [6].

Digital Health Records Smart hospitals adopt electronic health records (EHRs) and electronic medical records (EMRs) to digitise patient data. This enables easy access to patient information by healthcare providers and reduces paperwork, leading to more efficient care delivery.

Table 10.2 Summary table of EMRAM levels of technology adoption

European EMR Adoption Model	
Stage	Cumulative capabilities
0	Absence of basic systems
1	Three basic electronic systems installed (laboratory, radiology and pharmacy information)
2	Presence of a clinical data repository or electronic patient record
3	Clinical and nursing documentation may have clinical decision support for error checking during order entry
4	CPOE (computerised provider order entry—electronic instructions) in at least one clinical service area and/or for medication prescribing
5	Full complement of PACS (picture/image archiving system) replaces all film-based radiological images
6	Clinician documentation system which interacts with a clinical decision support tool and closed loop medication administration
7	Complete EMR and data continuity across services

IoT-Enabled Devices IoT devices, such as wearable health monitors, smart beds, and medical sensors, are used to collect real-time patient data. This data can be analysed to monitor patient health, detect abnormalities, and trigger alerts when necessary. It also helps service managers and ward nurses know where various resources, assets and medical equipment and devices are located at any given time through the use of real time location tracking.

Remote Monitoring and Telemedicine Smart hospitals use remote monitoring devices and telemedicine platforms to allow for virtual consultations, remote patient monitoring, and timely interventions. This is particularly valuable for managing chronic conditions and providing care in rural or underserved areas, as well as cutting down on out-patient attendance and it helps to maximise bed utilisation through virtual wards as seen in Chap. 3. Within the Hospital, remote monitoring technology is used for tracking patient status, early identification of the worsening of vital signs to prevent deterioration, detecting and reducing falls, identifying wandering patients, and facilitating greater insights into patient flow through the facility.

Automation and Robotics Automation technologies and robots are employed for various tasks, such as medication dispensing, surgery assistance, and repetitive administrative tasks, freeing up healthcare professionals to focus on patient care. Automated medication dispensing systems and barcoding technology help reduce medication errors and enhance medication management (Fig. 10.4).

Artificial Intelligence in Diagnostics AI is used for image analysis, diagnosis assistance, and treatment planning. AI algorithms can process vast amounts of med-

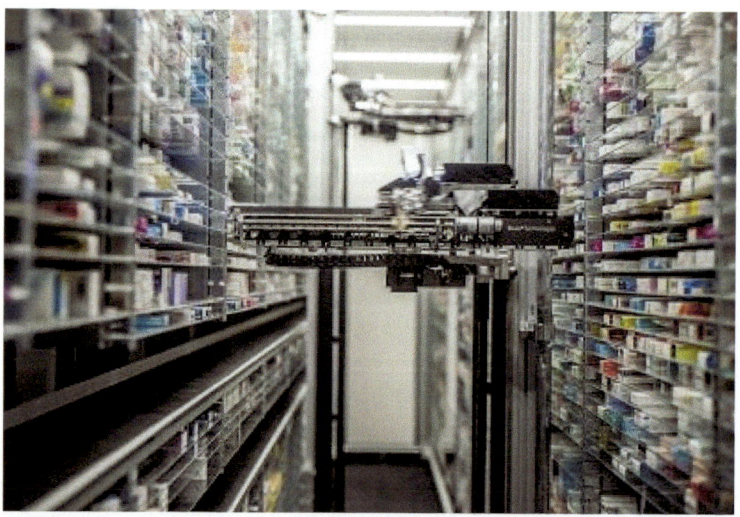

Fig. 10.4 A robotic pharmacy in action. Source: Rowa Technologies https://rowa.de/en/products/store-pick/ (unmodified). Courtesy and © Becton, Dickinson and Company

ical data to aid healthcare providers in making accurate diagnoses and treatment decisions. Artificial intelligence and machine learning algorithms can also be used for predictive analytics, diagnosis assistance, treatment planning, and personalised medicine. They can analyse vast datasets to identify trends and patterns that may not be apparent to human healthcare providers.

Clinical Command Centre This is a centralised hub or nerve centre that uses technology to monitor, coordinate and optimise various aspects of patient care and Hospital operations. It can support patient flow throughout the facility, bed management, identify deteriorating patients and use analytics to develop insights about the inner workings of the healthcare facility. Operational dashboards benefit from a digital twin representation of the whole hospital (patients, staff, assets) and allow a small team of clinically experienced professionals to run the Hospital like a form of air traffic control system. A clinical command centre (CCC) reflects the digital transformation of healthcare organisations, where advanced digital solutions are harnessed to improve operational efficiency, enhance patient care, and respond effectively to the dynamic healthcare landscape. The CCC is a central component of the digital hospital ecosystem, supporting a more connected and data-driven approach to healthcare delivery.

Energy Efficiency Hospitals consume on average twice as much energy as commercial buildings that are the same size. Smart hospitals prioritise energy efficiency by using smart building systems, renewable energy sources, and energy-saving technologies. This not only reduces operational costs but also contributes to environmental sustainability. Sensors are used to monitor environmental factors such as air quality, temperature, and humidity to maintain a safe and comfortable environment for patients and staff.

What Are the Benefits of Smart Hospitals?

Through the utilisation of various digital solutions, smart hospitals aim to improve patient outcomes, enhance the patient experience, reduce healthcare costs, and increase the efficiency of healthcare delivery. While the integration of technology offers many benefits, it also presents challenges related to data security, interoperability, and the need for ongoing staff training and adaptation to new technologies.

Patient safety is a key advantage and avoiding human error is vital. Smart hospitals use technology to enhance patient safety, such as fall detection systems, patient tracking, and medication error prevention mechanisms. In addition, optimisation of how a Hospital runs day to day (and over the longer term) is important to understand. Advanced scheduling systems and workflow optimisation tools help hospital staff manage patient flow, allocate resources efficiently, and reduce wait times. Big data analytics are used to analyse healthcare trends, outcomes, and costs, enabling data-driven decision-making and continuous improvement in healthcare delivery.

Allied to this are the opportunities for research and innovation—smart hospitals often serve as hubs for medical research and new developments, facilitating collaboration among researchers and healthcare providers both locally and globally to advance medical knowledge and treatment options.

In terms of the resources required to run a Hospital and the management of facilities, smart hospitals employ data analytics to optimise inventory management, reducing waste and ensuring that essential supplies are readily available. Energy-efficient building systems, lighting, and HVAC (heating, ventilation, and air conditioning) systems reduce operational costs and the hospital's environmental footprint. In terms of predictive maintenance, IoT sensors can be used to monitor the condition of medical equipment and the Hospital infrastructure, enabling early repairs or building 'self-healing' to reduce downtime and ensure the reliability of critical systems.

The ultimate benefits of a smart Hospital might be summarised as two-fold, firstly to increase the overall efficiency of delivering a complex system. Secondly, and more humanly it is about patient engagement and quality of care. Smart hospitals use technology to shift the focus onto engaging patients in their own care, making things more accessible, convenient and user friendly. This includes patient portals, mobile apps, and educational resources to help patients make informed decisions about their health and to improve the still relatively scary experience of having to come in to a Hospital.

What Are the Challenges Faced by Smart Hospitals?

Smart hospitals, while promising in their potential to improve healthcare delivery, face several challenges that must be addressed for their successful implementation and operation.

Some of the key issues include high implementation costs—the upfront costs associated with the adoption of advanced technologies and infrastructure can be substantial (and eye-watering for the uninitiated). This includes the expense of purchasing and implementing electronic health records, IoT devices, and AI systems as well as the ongoing operating costs which need to be absorbed into business as usual. Balancing the allocation of resources between technology investments and direct patient care can be a delicate process, as investments in technology can be resource intensive. Integration with existing infrastructure, many hospitals have legacy systems in place, and integrating new technologies with existing infrastructure can be complex and costly. Ensuring that the technology infrastructure remains up to date and functions optimally over time requires ongoing maintenance and investment, both in terms of hardware and software updates.

From a technical perspective interoperability can be a major blocker. Integrating various technologies and systems within a hospital can be complex. Lack of standardised protocols and interfaces can hinder interoperability between different healthcare systems and devices, making data sharing and integration difficult. Therefore, ensuring that different devices and software can communicate and share data seamlessly is a significant challenge. Additionally, data security and privacy are relevant concerns—smart hospitals deal with vast amounts of sensitive patient data, making them attractive targets for cyberattacks. Ensuring robust cybersecurity measures and compliance with data protection regulations is crucial to safeguard patient information. Testing the reliability of critical systems is essential, as downtime can have life-threatening consequences. Implementing backup systems and disaster recovery plans is crucial. As technology evolves, smart hospitals must plan for scalability to accommodate future growth and changing healthcare needs. This includes anticipating increases in patient volumes and data storage requirements.

Service users must have confidence in the security and ethical use of their data. Obtaining informed consent for data collection and sharing while maintaining patient trust is challenging and if there are high numbers of people opting out then it can affect the effective of the overall system. While smart hospitals aim to engage patients in their care, not all patients may be tech-savvy or have access to the necessary tools. Ensuring inclusivity and accessibility for all patient populations can be challenging (more on this in the next chapter).

Smart hospitals must navigate a complex landscape of healthcare regulations and standards. Ensuring compliance with local, national, and international regulations is essential. Collecting vast amounts of healthcare data is only valuable if it can be effectively analysed and translated into actionable insights. Managing and interpreting this data can be challenging.

Ethical and legal concerns—the use of AI in diagnostics and treatment decisions raises ethical and legal questions, particularly regarding accountability for medical errors and the delegation of responsibilities to automated systems. Determining liability in cases of medical errors or data breaches involving smart hospital technologies can be legally complex and contentious.

Finally, there is the issue of staff training and resistance to change. Not all healthcare professionals and Hospital managers have the capabilities to use new and complex systems, so a significant amount of work needs to be done around upskilling. Healthcare professionals may also resist adopting new technologies because of the dislike of change and a reliance on sticking with old ways of working. There can be a learning curve associated with using these systems. Providing adequate training and addressing resistance to change are essential.

Addressing these challenges requires collaboration among healthcare providers, technology vendors, regulatory bodies, and policymakers. It also involves ongoing evaluation and adaptation of strategies to ensure that smart hospitals effectively and ethically improve healthcare delivery while mitigating the risks and challenges (new smart hospital design standards are summarised in Table 10.3 below).

Table 10.3 Summary overview of the design principles/standards for new smart/digital hospitals

SMART HOSPITAL STANDARDS—2024
New technologies and systems should comply with the following.

INTEROPERABILITY	Digital systems must integrate and communicate effectively with one another. Enforcement of interoperability standards and the elimination of proprietary systems (wherever possible) is essential.
COMPLIANCE	Hospital technologies must meet all relevant international regulatory standards.
DATA SECURITY	Data privacy and information governance need to be effectively built in to Hospital systems and tested and updated on a regular basis.
CLINICAL SAFETY	Digital solutions should be focused on eliminating known sources of clinical error whilst at the same time they must be evaluated and mitigated to ensure that new problems do not arise that could be harmful to patient care.
USER-FRIENDLY	Increasingly complex systems should be designed with end-users in mind and only implemented if they meet specific usability criteria for Hospital staff and patients.
CARE QUALITY	Technologies are an enabler of improvements in care delivery, so they must have clearly realisable benefits for patients and healthcare professionals.
SCALBILITY/ FLEXIBILITY	As hospitals grow, services expand and patient needs change over time, technologies should be implemented with flexibility in mind to ensure future proofing.
SUSTAINABILITY	Hospitals are energy intensive facilities thus environmentally friendly operations need to be considered for all new smart developments.

Summary

Smart Hospitals build on the foundation of digital technologies and comprise a set of interconnected technologies that form the central nervous system or neural network of a healthcare system. The sharing of data from numerous sources allows this network to monitor and react to feedback, learn and grow in an emergent fashion. The goal is to provide better patient care delivery, through better operational processes and flow, within a well organised and future proofed infrastructure. Centralising such technologies as a focus for data collection and sharing also acts as a harmonious node for virtual care delivery.

For existing hospitals, doing nothing is not an option. They need to integrate new digital health technologies in a phased manner, redesign how they are delivering all forms of care, consider how they network with other health and social care organisations, and shift functions that can be outsourced to others who can perform them more cost effectively and efficiently. Whilst it is important to harness the benefits of digital solutions in a smart Hospital it is crucial that every input is connected to the ultimate goal of improved patient care delivery.

References

1. Asan Medical Center. A paradigm shift initiated by experience. https://news-en.amc.seoul.kr/news/eng/detail.do?cntId=2795
2. Kwon H, An S, Lee HY, et al. Review of smart hospital services in real healthcare environments. Healthc Inform Res. 2022;28(1):3–15. https://doi.org/10.4258/hir.2022.28.1.3.
3. O'Brien C. New children's hospital to break fresh ground in digital healthcare. Irish Times. 2023 Feb. https://www.irishtimes.com/business/2023/02/02/new-childrens-hospital-to-break-fresh-ground-in-digital-healthcare/
4. Cleveland Clinic Abu Dhabi ranked no.1 smart hospital in the UAE and GCC by Newsweek. https://www.clevelandclinicabudhabi.ae/en/media-center/news/cleveland-clinic-abu-dhabi-ranked-no-1-smart-hospital-in-the-uae-and-gcc-by-newsweek
5. Patient first: how Karolinska University Hospital is transforming to meet future demands of healthcare. https://www.philips.se/a-w/about/news/archive/standard/case-studies/20190128-patient-first-how-karolinska-university-hospital-is-transforming-to-meet-future-demands-of-healthcare.html
6. HIMSS. Digital health transformation. https://www.himss.org/what-we-do-solutions/digital-health-transformation/maturity-models/electronic-medical-record-adoption-model-emram

Further Reading

Day S, Zweig M. 2018 year end funding report: is digital health in a bubble? Rock Health.
OECD iLibrary. Digital health at a glance. https://www.oecd-ilibrary.org/sites/7a7afb35-en/1/3/2/index.html?itemId=/content/publication/7a7afb35-en&_csp_=6cf33e24b6584414b81774026d82a571&itemIGO=oecd&itemContentType=book#

Chapter 11
Algorithmic Medicine

Abstract This chapter explores the profound impact of algorithms, AI, machine learning and data analytics on modern healthcare. As the digital transformation of medicine continues to evolve, the integration of algorithms into medical practice is redefining how we interact with patients, how we choose and interpret diagnostics, plan treatment, and deliver patient care. We delve into the key applications, benefits, challenges, and ethical considerations surrounding algorithmic medicine, shedding light on the dynamic intersection of healthcare and potential 'black box' technology.

Keywords Medical algorithms · Rules engines · Clinical pathways · Clinical decision support · Artificial intelligence · Machine learning · Clinical risk management · Medical ethics

Defining Algorithmic Medicine

An algorithm simply takes one set of inputs and through a group of pre-determined rules produces some form of output. The important consideration here is what exactly those rules are, how many of them are there, what they are contingent on, who wrote them, did they have all the right information, are they the right rules, have they been validated, are they universally applicable and most importantly, are they safe? In fact, the concept of algorithms themselves generates so much discussion and ire that there are whole sections of the internet dedicated to their fallacies and dangers.

An example of an algorithmic approach to medical care is anything from body mass index (BMI) calculation (the relationship between your body weight and height), to decision trees for the management of acute chest pain and pathways for the selection of the best medication for an agitated patient (see Fig. 11.1 below).

Proponents of AI in medicine are usually not shy about pointing out the flaws of clinicians, such as their susceptibility to cognitive biases and to committing diagnostic errors. Medical decision-making involves high degrees of uncertainty and clinicians are prone to reasoning errors.

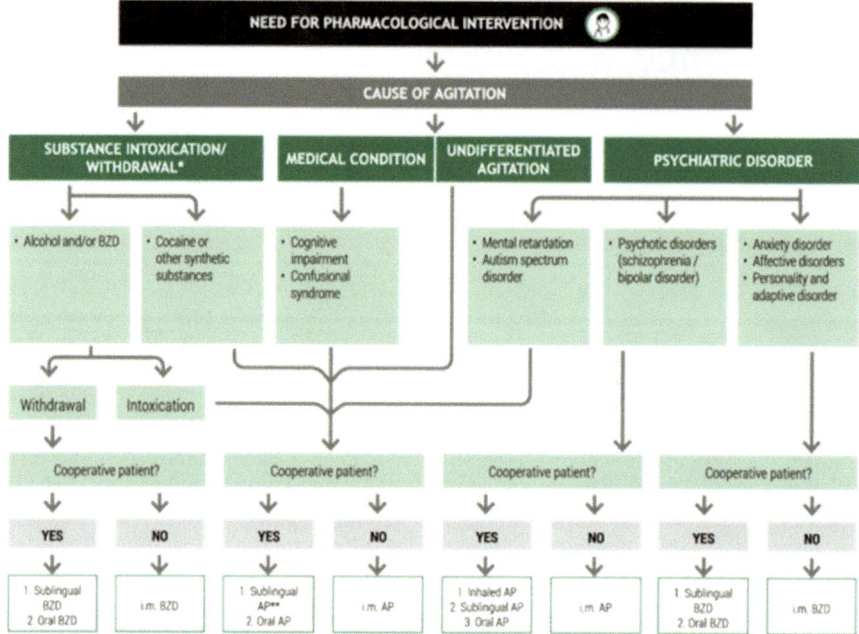

Fig. 11.1 Example algorithmic flow for management of patients with psychomotor agitation. Reproduced from Vieta et al. (2017) [1]. Reproduced under Creative Commons licence. The Creative Commons Public Domain Dedication waiver (http://creativecommons.org/publicdomain/zero/1.0/) applies to the data made available in this article, unless otherwise stated

The idea of using an algorithm to manage an unwell patient has its roots in various fields, including medicine, computer science, and artificial intelligence. Patients and clinicians face shared clinical decision-making tasks while under time constraints and high cognitive loads from large volumes of information. Here are some key developments and influences that have contributed to the use of algorithms in healthcare:

Evidence Based Medicine This involves using the best available evidence from scientific research to inform clinical decision-making. Algorithms play a role in synthesising, grading and analysing this evidence, then helping healthcare providers apply it appropriately, matching research findings to both clinical guideline creation and individual patient cases. One of the subsequent aims is then to use this evidence to standardise medical treatments and reduce variation in the way that people and populations are cared for.

Clinical Decision Support Systems (CDSS) Specialised software designed to assist healthcare professionals in making clinical decisions by providing relevant information at the point of care. Early systems used rule-based algorithms to analyse patient data and offer recommendations based on common or likely scenarios. For example, Yale and Mayo clinic produced a specialist application for the assessment of patients with head injuries [2]. The software incorporated the latest clinical guidelines and helped to evaluate the severity of the injury. By using these two strands, the system was able to reduce the number of CT head scans that were being undertaken. Clinicians often tend to err on the side of caution and request scans that aren't indicated, so the use of such a system facilitates both safe and more appropriate assessment strategies. Other use cases for a CDSS (which may also be incorporated into an electronic patient record) include performing calculations for drug dosing, the triggering of reminders or alerts and analysing the severity of blood test results in order to prompt intervention.

Artificial Intelligence in Medicine The integration of AI into medicine has significantly influenced the use of algorithms in patient management. One smart system designed and developed at Vanderbilt University in Nashville used a host of patient information including age, gender, postcode, medical history, admissions data and medication, to predict suicide risk in their cohort of patients [3]. They based their algorithm on data collected from 5000 admissions of patients who has been brought to Hospital for self-harm or attempted suicide. The algorithm was able to predict with 84% accuracy whether someone would subsequently attempt suicide within 1 week and was 80% accurate at suicide prediction within the next 2 years.

Similarly, researchers at the University of Nottingham created an algorithm which scans the routine medical data of patients and is able to calculate which of them are at high risk of having a stroke or heart attack within the next 10 years (this early flagging allowing preventative measures to be put in place) [4]. When compared with the standard approach to predicting cardiovascular risk the AI system was able to correctly predict outcomes for 355 more patients. Dr. Stephen Weng who led on the research said, "*AI medical tools being tested today will soon boost clinicians' accuracy in both diagnosis and prognosis*" [5].

The use of AI for pattern recognition in medical diagnostics has also seen significant progress. AI algorithms are being used to improve the accuracy and speed of testing processes in radiology, pathology, and cardiology. This includes AI-driven image recognition for early detection of diseases like breast and skin cancer and there have been examples of AI systems outperforming human radiologists in the identification of malignant disease.

Machine learning algorithms, a subset of AI, can analyse large datasets to identify patterns and make predictions (Fig. 11.2). This capability is valuable for diagnosing diseases, predicting patient outcomes, and personalising treatment plans. HCA Healthcare have created a Sepsis Prediction algorithm for their Hospital chain. Based on experience developed from large data sets it constantly scans and monitors patient data (such a pulse, blood pressure and temperature readings) to pick up signs of sepsis (generalised infection) at an early stage—approximately 6 hours sooner than would normally be the case—and more accurately than clinicians. This can automatically alert the Hospital's intensive care outreach teams (rapid response clinicians) and guides them through the steps that need to be taken to avert deterioration and prevent complications. According to a report in the Wall Street Journal this has led to an impressive reduction in mortality of 30% across 160 Hospitals [7].

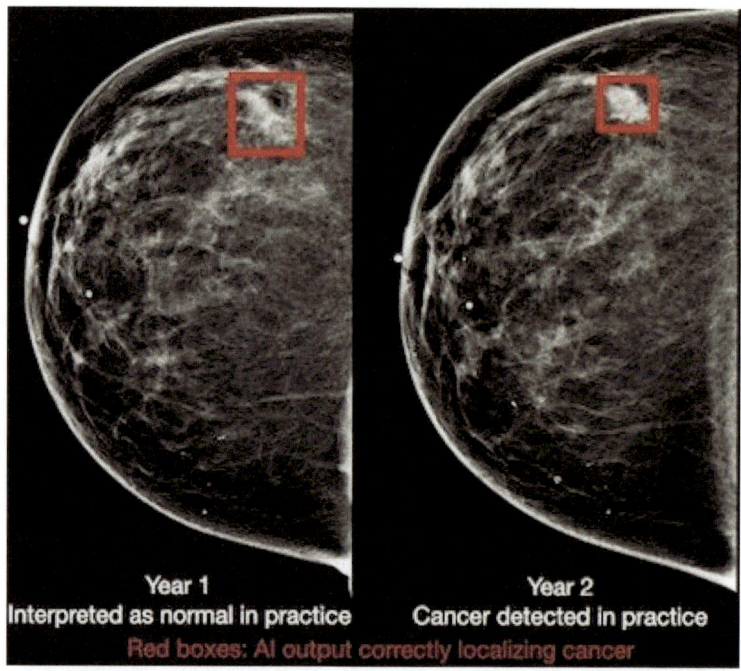

Fig. 11.2 AI software is often able to detect changes associated with malignancy before human operators. Reproduced with permissions from Lotter et al. (2021) [6]

Natural Language Processing (NLP) for Healthcare NLP is a form of machine learning which enables the processing and analysis of free text. NLP algorithms are being used to analyse medical records, clinical notes, and patient-Doctor interactions. They help extract valuable insights, support clinical decision-making, and improve the accuracy of medical coding. It can aid in the prediction of patient outcomes, augment hospital triage systems, and generate diagnostic models that detect early-stage chronic disease.

NLP has the capability to facilitate natural language generation (NLG), allowing patients to effectively communicate with chatbots and obtain pertinent information by asking questions. Large language models have been trained on massive datasets. An example is MedPaLM which has been designed to respond to health and disease related questions from patients and the general public, by encoding clinical knowledge and using data about medical conditions and their associated findings. This is still undergoing evaluation but has the potential to act as a medical equivalent to ChatGPT. Given the concerns about accuracy and safety in a medical context, it's roll out to end-users may be some way off. An example of the instruction prompt tuning for MedPaLM is shown below in Box 11.1.

> **Box 11.1 Example of an Instruction Prompt for a Medical Decision Support Tool**
> **You are a helpful medical knowledge assistant. Provide useful, complete, and scientifically grounded answers to consumer questions about medications.**
>
> **Question:** How can I split a 3 mg or 4 mg warfarin pill so I can get a 2.5 mg pill?
>
> **Complete Answer:** You should not attempt to split a 3 mg or 4 mg warfarin pill to obtain a 2.5 mg dose. If you are prescribed warfarin in a 2.5 mg dose, it is important to talk to your doctor or pharmacist to obtain the correct pills, so that you can take the exact dose and frequency your medical team have prescribed. Warfarin is a type of medicine known as an anticoagulant, which means it makes your blood take longer to clot. The exact amount required to achieve the desired effect can vary.

There are challenges to the use of NLP in medicine. The underlying data on which a system is trained on should be unbiased. This is an essential requirement if the conclusions reached or suggestions made by NLP algorithms are to be trusted. Healthcare professionals will be required to undergo training in order to effectively utilise natural language processing (NLP) as a safe tool in their regular practice. In the near future, NLP technology is expected to be seamlessly integrated into the clinical setting, working alongside clinicians to generate problem lists, provide patient-oriented applications for efficient triage processes, and serve as a valuable resource for analysing extensive amounts of unstructured data. This has the potential to greatly enhance personalised and timely evidence-based medicine practices.

Drug Discovery and Repurposing Algorithms are playing a crucial role in drug discovery, accelerating the identification of potential drug candidates, which traditionally takes many years and billions of dollars to complete. Scientists can utilise AI to pinpoint the precise proteins or molecular pathways implicated in disease and subsequently create medications that specifically target these proteins or pathways. This approach can effectively lower the risk of unintended effects and enhance the safety and effectiveness of drugs. AI-driven algorithms are also being used to repurpose existing drugs for new medical applications (see Fig. 11.3 below).

Personalised Medicine Algorithmic approaches are being employed to develop personalised treatment plans. Genomic data, in particular, is used to match patients with treatments tailored to their genetic makeup and individual medical history.

Most practitioners use only a small segment of algorithmic medicine routinely. Arguably however, there is a growing need for algorithms in healthcare as the volume of medical data increases, as well as the increasing demand on clinicians. The intended goal of using an algorithm is to improve and standardise care—enabling

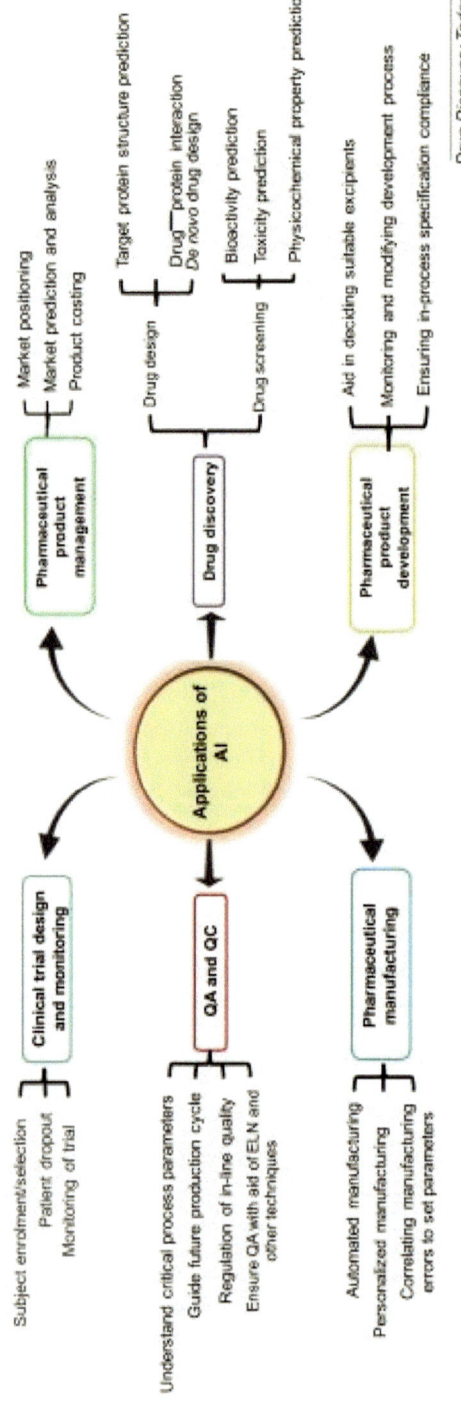

Fig. 11.3 Drug discovery applications of Artifical Intelligence. Reproduced with permissions from Paul et al. 2021 [8]

the implementation of best practice and the reduction of variation (one of the most problematic aspects of current medical care). Currently the outputs of manual or automated algorithms (many of which are presented as protocols) are reviewed and approved by clinicians—who can temper raw information with their skill, clinical experience and practical wisdom.

Concerns and Risk Reduction Regarding AI in Medicine

The majority of what we hear about AI pushes a positive agenda about the future of medicine, but of course, algorithms can be wrong or produce unexpected results and AI has the potential to fail. Following an algorithm can be a valuable and efficient approach in many situations, but there are also potential problems and limitations associated with relying solely on algorithms without thinking and interpretation. Some of the common issues include:

Lack of Flexibility Algorithms are designed to follow a specific set of instructions. They may not adapt well to unexpected or novel situations, and human intervention or judgment may be necessary to address such cases.

Assumption of Data Quality There is a common assumption that input data is accurate and reliable. If the data used to feed an algorithm is flawed or biased, it can lead to incorrect results or decisions. Algorithms can perpetuate biases present in their training data, leading to unfair or discriminatory outcomes, particularly in areas like hiring, lending, or law enforcement and killer robots.

Overfitting In machine learning, overfitting can occur when an algorithm is trained too closely on a specific dataset, resulting in poor generalisation to new data (or a different population set with different characteristics). Algorithms may struggle to understand context or nuances, making them less effective in tasks that require a deep understanding of human language, culture, or complex social dynamics.

Lack of Ethical Judgment Algorithms cannot make moral or ethical decisions. In some situations, making purely algorithmic decisions can be ethically problematic [9].

Data Privacy Concerns Algorithms often require access to sensitive data, raising concerns about confidentiality and security. Unauthorised access or data breaches can lead to significant issues.

Maintenance and Updates Algorithms require maintenance and updates to remain effective. Failure to refresh algorithms can result in outdated, inefficient, or insecure systems.

Human Resistance In some cases, human users may resist following algorithms, especially if they perceive them as intrusive, limiting, or undermining their expertise. We all know someone who refuses to follow their GPS for example. This is a challenge to the epistemic authority of clinicians, which may in turn lead to patterns of defensive medical practice, disagreements with decision making and ultimately lead to patient harm.

Complexity Some algorithms can be highly complex and challenging to understand, making them less accessible to those who need to use or interpret them, exacerbated by the black box phenomenon.

Reliability and Testing Ensuring the reliability and accuracy of an algorithm, particularly in critical applications like healthcare or autonomous vehicles, can be a significant challenge. Who is to be accountable at either an individual or an organisational level if an algorithm turns out to be flawed and systematically prescribing erroneous treatments? Healthcare systems may pressurise clinicians to use AI systems for the purposes of time and efficiency savings and they will be the ones who are culpable.

Interoperability When using multiple algorithms in a system, ensuring that they work together seamlessly can be complicated. Incompatibility between different algorithms can lead to inefficiencies and conflicts, especially if there are antagonistic end goals e.g. cost savings versus patient safety.

Resource Intensiveness Certain algorithms, especially in machine learning and deep learning, can be resource-intensive, requiring powerful hardware and significant computational resources.

Human Disengagement Excessive reliance on algorithms may lead to human disengagement or reduced accountability in decision-making processes.

Unforeseen Consequences Algorithms can have unintended consequences, particularly in complex and dynamic systems, which can be difficult to predict but not a surprise to fans of HAL in 2001.

The introduction and use of such systems therefore needs to be dealt with in accordance with our professional duties of care and caution about safety because the downside of a broken or inappropriate AI system is harm to patients and distrust in healthcare. A large part of the worry about machine learning and AI is due to the nature of its complexity, involving as they do, sophisticated and opaque mathematical relationships between the data inputs and the system outputs. This is exacerbated by the use of potentially biased, low quality or less relevant underlying datasets that the programmes are based on, and absent human control over the generation of predictions because they are coming from a black box. Melissa McCradden from the Department of Bioethics at the Hospital for Sick Children in Toronto believes that the current strategies being used for the evaluation of medical algorithms are poorly suited for what they are needed for, and they do not address the gap between intended and real-world performance of AI systems in the field of medicine [10].

Such concerns have led an international group of researchers, headed by Professor Alisatair Dennison and Dr. Lauren Oakden-Rayner, to develop a medical algorithm audit framework that can assess algorithms on the basis of potential errors in the context of a clinical task, mapping the components that might contribute to the occurrence of errors, and anticipating their potential consequences [11]. This tool can be used to better understand the weaknesses of an AI system and put in place mechanisms to mitigate their impact. The authors propose that safety monitoring and medical algorithmic auditing should be a joint responsibility between users and developers and encourage the use of feedback mechanisms between these groups to promote learning and maintain safe deployment of artificial intelligence systems.

The elements of the audit (shown in Fig. 11.4 below) include mapping the scope of the AI system and its intended use, assessing alignment to the intended clinical pathway and looking at the source data. Testing then needs to take place to explore for errors, test subgroups (to check for relevance) and adversarial testing (to try and break the system). This is then followed by identification of risk mitigation measures and an iterative process with the developers. This is something that could potentially be reinforced through the clinical evaluation sign off process that notified bodies have to undertake when certifying new medical devices and software.

Ideal algorithms in health care need to be explainable (the significance of features in determining outputs can be effectively communicated by evaluating their relative importance), dynamic (i.e. updatable when the evidence changes), precise, autonomous (learn with minimal supervision and execute without human input), fair (evaluate and mitigate implicit bias and social inequity) and reproducible (validated externally and shared with academic communities for scrutiny) according to Tyler Loftus and colleagues from the University of Florida, so as to allow the maximum potential benefits to patients and clinicians (see Fig. 11.5 below) [12].

Addressing the problems of algorithmic medicine requires a careful approach. While algorithms are valuable tools, it's essential to use them in conjunction with human judgment and expertise, regularly update and assess their performance, and ensure transparency and fairness in their application. Ethical considerations and data quality are particularly important in algorithmic decision-making, as they can significantly impact the outcomes and consequences of their use.

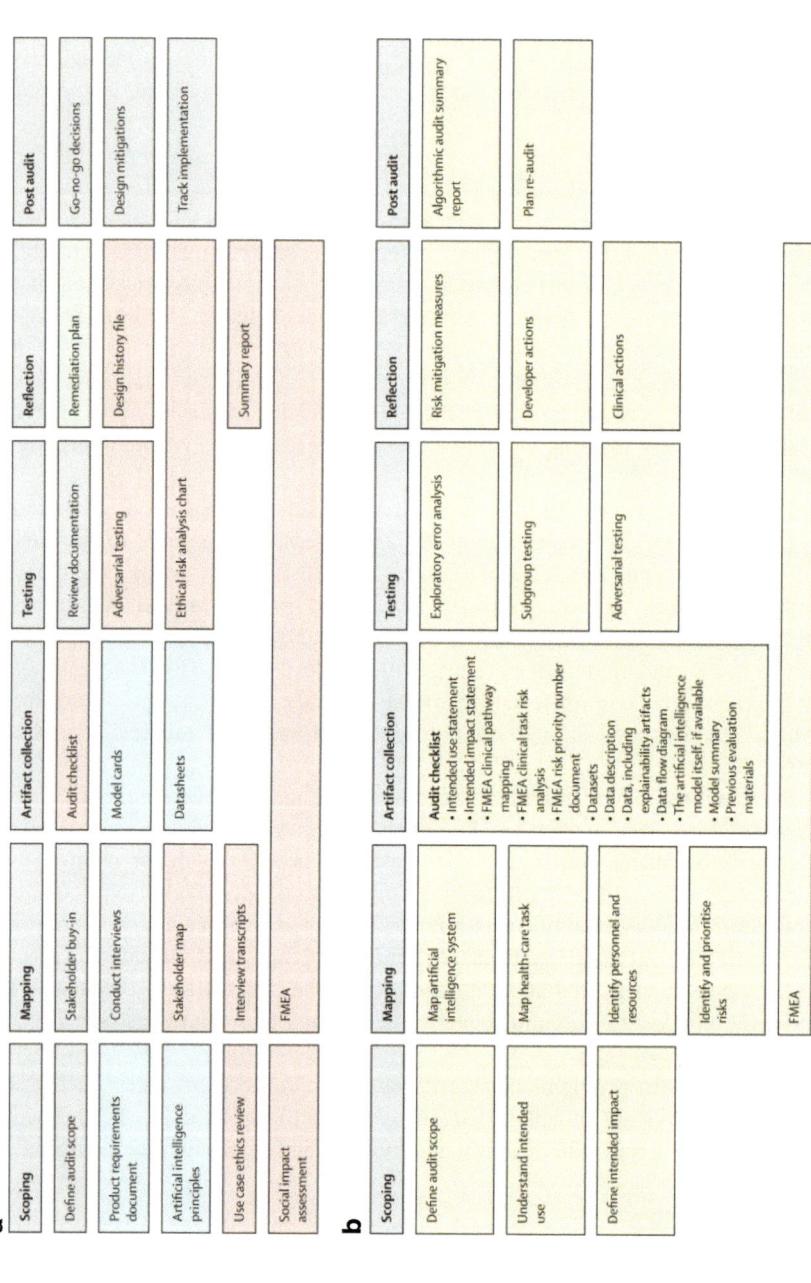

Fig. 11.4 Medical algorithm two part audit framework. Reproduced with permissions from Liu et al. 2022 [11] (https://www.thelancet.com/journals/landig/article/PIIS2589-7500%2822%2900003-6/fulltext#figures unmodified)

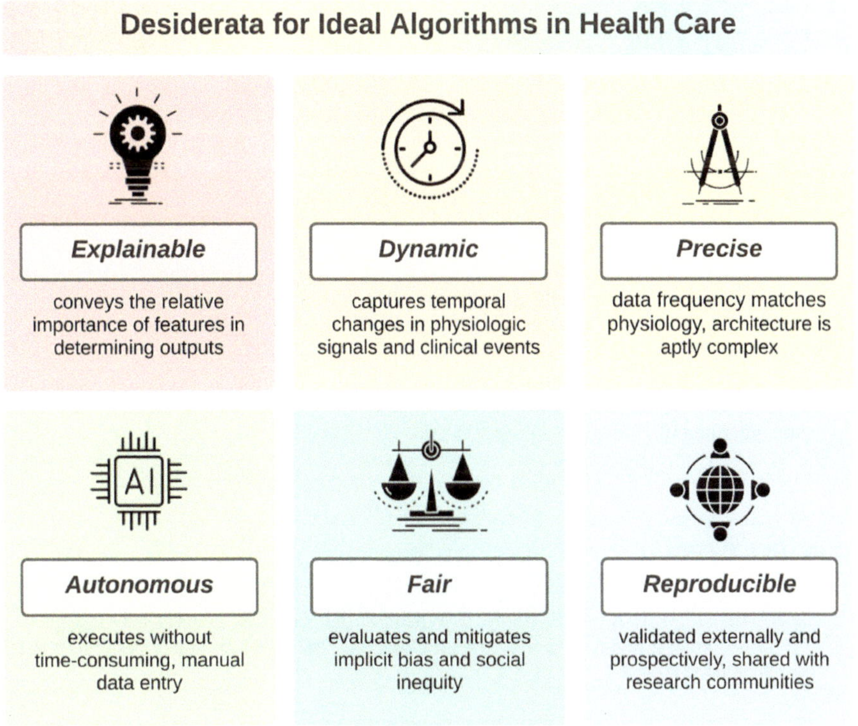

Desiderata for Ideal Algorithms in Health Care

Explainable

conveys the relative importance of features in determining outputs

Dynamic

captures temporal changes in physiologic signals and clinical events

Precise

data frequency matches physiology, architecture is aptly complex

Autonomous

executes without time-consuming, manual data entry

Fair

evaluates and mitigates implicit bias and social inequity

Reproducible

validated externally and prospectively, shared with research communities

Fig. 11.5 Overview of aspects to consider when assessing medical algorithms. Reproduced from Loftus et al. 2022 [12] under Creative Commons Licence 4.0. https://creativecommons.org/licenses/by/4.0/

References

1. Vieta E, Garriga M, Cardete L, et al. Protocol for the management of psychiatric patients with psychomotor agitation. BMC Psychiatry. 2017;17:328. https://doi.org/10.1186/s12888-017-1490-0.
2. Ballard DW, Kuppermann N, Vinson DR, et al.; Pediatric Emergency Care Applied Research Network (PECARN); Clinical Research on Emergency Services and Treatment (CREST) Network; Partners HealthCare. Implementation of a clinical decision support system for children with minor blunt head trauma who are at nonnegligible risk for traumatic brain injuries. Ann Emerg Med. 2019;73(5):440–51. https://doi.org/10.1016/j.annemergmed.2018.11.011.
3. Walsh CG, Ribeiro JD, Franklin JC. Predicting risk of suicide attempts over time through machine learning. Clin Psychol Sci. 2017;5(3):457–69. https://doi.org/10.1177/2167702617691560.
4. Weng SF, Vaz L, Qureshi N, Kai J. Prediction of premature all-cause mortality: a prospective general population cohort study comparing machine-learning and standard epidemiological approaches. PLoS One. 2019;14(3):e0214365. https://doi.org/10.1371/journal.pone.0214365.
5. Strickland E. AI predicts heart attacks and strokes more accurately than standard doctor's method. IEEE Spectrum. https://spectrum.ieee.org/ai-predicts-heart-attacks-more-accurately-than-standard-doctor-method#:~:text=Weng%20says%20the%20AI%20medical,that%20look%20like%20in%20practice%3F

6. Lotter W, Diab AR, Haslam B, et al. Robust breast cancer detection in mammography and digital breast tomosynthesis using an annotation-efficient deep learning approach. Nat Med. 2021;27:244–9. https://doi.org/10.1038/s41591-020-01174-9.

7. Landro L. How hospitals are using AI to save lives. Wall Street Journal. 2022 Apr. https://www.wsj.com/articles/how-hospitals-are-using-ai-to-save-lives-11649610000.

8. Paul D, Sanap G, Shenoy S, Kalyane D, Kalia K, Tekade RK. Artificial intelligence in drug discovery and development. Drug Discov Today. 2021;26(1):80–93. https://doi.org/10.1016/j.drudis.2020.10.010.

9. Grote T, Berens P. On the ethics of algorithmic decision-making in healthcare. J Med Ethics. 2020;46:205–11.

10. McCradden MD, Stephenson EA, Anderson JA. Clinical research underlies ethical integration of healthcare artificial intelligence. Nat Med. 2020;26:1325–6.

11. Liu X, Glocker B, McCradden MM, Ghassemi M, Denniston AK, Oakden-Rayner L. The medical algorithmic audit. Lancet Digit Health. 2022;4:e384–97.

12. Loftus TJ, Tighe PJ, Ozrazgat-Baslanti T, et al. Ideal algorithms in healthcare: explainable, dynamic, precise, autonomous, fair, and reproducible. PLOS Digit Health. 2022;1(1):e0000006. https://doi.org/10.1371/journal.pdig.0000006.

Further Reading

Locke S, Bashall A, Al-Adely S, Moore J, Wilson A, Kitchen GB. Natural language processing in medicine: a review. Trends Anaesth Crit Care. 2021;38:4–9. https://doi.org/10.1016/j.tacc.2021.02.007.

Chapter 12
The Digitally Excluded Patient

Abstract In the ever-evolving landscape of healthcare, the integration of digital technologies has become increasingly pervasive. Electronic health records, telemedicine, mobile health apps, and wearable devices have transformed the way healthcare is delivered and accessed. However, amid this digital revolution, a significant portion of the patient population remains digitally excluded. This chapter explores the multifaceted phenomenon of the digitally excluded patient, shedding light on the challenges and opportunities this presents in the context of modern healthcare. By delving into the factors that contribute to digital exclusion, we gain a deeper understanding of the barriers that impede patient access to digital health tools and information. As well as examining the impact on patient outcomes, healthcare disparities, and the patient-provider relationship, we should also highlight the ethical considerations surrounding digital healthcare, emphasising the importance of equity and inclusivity in the digital age.

Keywords Digital inclusion · Digital exclusion · Remote and rural medicine · Internet accessibility · Digital divide · Digital health · Smartphone usage

Navigating Healthcare in a Digital World

The digitalisation of healthcare has ushered in a new era of medical advances and improved accessibility which hopes to empower patients and their carers. However, as healthcare systems and services become increasingly reliant on technology, a significant portion of the patient population remain on the outside of this. This chapter explores the challenges and consequences faced by digitally excluded patients and delves into strategies for mitigating the digital divide in healthcare and ways of enhancing the digital literacy of service users.

Digital inclusion relates to whether individuals have the equipment, skills and literacy to be able to use connected devices such as smartphones, tablets and the internet, along with the connectivity (the right infrastructure of broadband, WiFi or mobile) and access to digital services (which includes usability). Recent figures

P. Grant, *The Virtual Hospital*, https://doi.org/10.1007/978-3-031-69944-3_12

suggest that 90% of households have internet access and 78% of people go online using a mobile device. 54% of people have looked up health information online in a 3-month period and 9% of adults have a smart watch or fitness tracker [1]. The benefits of being online are social, financial, health and wellbeing related and 77% of people believe that internet access is now an essential need. Medical services working through various technological routes need to be accessible. Table 12.1 represents a commonly used scale of inclusion relating to internet use, from 1 to 9.

Digital exclusion essentially means the opposite. It's the situation where certain individuals or groups are unable to access, use, or benefit from digital technologies and the internet. It represents a lack of participation or inclusion in the digital society and is often associated with disparities in access to technology, digital skills, and online opportunities. Digital exclusion can manifest in various forms and can affect different demographics, including low-income communities, elderly individuals, people with disabilities, and those living in remote or underserved areas.

The Consumer Digital Index [2] shows:

- 11.9 million people (22% of the population) do not have the digital skills needed for everyday life in the UK.
- One-third of the offline struggle to interact with healthcare services.
- By 2030 it is predicted that 4.5 million people (8% of the population) will remain digitally disengaged.
- People with a disability are 35% less likely to have the essential digital skills for life.

In the United States, 24 million people lack access to high-speed internet, and many more cannot connect due to gaps in digital equity and literacy [3]. The inability to use the internet pushes access to many essential services out of reach. Often, this compounds other inequities and historical injustices.

The Digital Divide In developed countries, there are demographic and regional inequalities in digital engagement. Digital approaches can have unintended consequences, such as excluding those who are less digitally literate or who do not have access to the most advanced telecommunication services. It will take focus to ensure the push for digital ways of working can help tackle these health inequalities rather

Table 12.1 Scale of digital inclusion

Digital inclusion scale (use of the internet)	
1	Never have, never will
2	Was online, but no longer
3	Willing and unable
4	Reluctantly online
5	Learning the ropes
6	Task specific
7	Basic digital skills
8	Confident
9	Expert

than exacerbate them. In an increasingly digital world, people who are digitally excluded are at risk of worse access to services and worse health outcomes. People with the greatest health needs are also often the most at risk of being left behind and building digital services with this in mind, we need to ensure high levels of accessibility.

During the COVID-19 lockdowns, the restrictions on social contact and mobility meant that many people with mental health problems (such as severe depression, schizophrenia, bipolar disorder and psychosis) and those receiving community mental health rehabilitation were unable to get the access to services and support that they desperately required [4]. In many services there was a shift to digital delivery using telemedicine as a way of providing care and consultations online. People affected by the digital divide were disproportionately limited because they couldn't access such services, and this will have compounded the severity and extent of their psychiatric problems. The global risks report from the World Economic Forum in 2021 exposed the extent of the digital divide, with 60% of adults being found to lack the digital skills required to work, learn and access critical services online [5]. It's really important that post-pandemic healthcare services used by people with serious mental health problems should focus on both facilitating digital engagement and continuing to offer non-digital alternatives for those not yet able to engage with digital services.

Characteristics of the Digitally Excluded

Lack of Access to Technology Individuals who do not have access to essential digital tools such as computers, smartphones, or tablets may experience digital exclusion. This lack of access can be due to economic constraints, limited infrastructure, or geographical factors.

Limited Internet Connectivity Access to high-speed and reliable internet is crucial for participating in the digital world. Digital exclusion can occur when individuals or communities lack access to affordable and reliable internet services.

Digital Skills Gap Digital exclusion is often linked to a lack of digital literacy and skills. Individuals who are not familiar with using computers, navigating the internet, or using digital applications may find it challenging to engage in online activities, or be fearful or reluctant.

Economic Barriers Affordability is a significant factor in digital exclusion. The cost of devices, internet services, and relevant software can be prohibitive for individuals or families with limited financial resources.

Language and Content Barriers Digital exclusion may occur when online content is not available in the languages spoken by certain communities. Additionally, individuals with limited literacy or those who speak languages not well-supported online may face challenges in accessing information.

Disabilities and Accessibility Issues   People with disabilities may experience digital exclusion if websites, applications, or digital content are not designed to be accessible. This includes issues related to visual, auditory, motor, or cognitive impairments.

Social and Cultural Factors   Digital exclusion can also be influenced by social and cultural dimensions. Some individuals or communities may be hesitant to embrace digital technologies due to cultural norms, privacy concerns, or a lack of perceived relevance.

Geographical Isolation   Individuals living in remote or rural areas may face challenges in accessing digital infrastructure, including high-speed internet, which can contribute to digital exclusion.

Addressing digital exclusion involves implementing strategies to overcome these barriers, such as providing affordable access to technology, offering digital literacy training, creating accessible online content, and developing inclusive policies. Bridging the digital divide is essential for promoting social equity, economic opportunities, and overall community development in an increasingly digital world. Innovative solutions and interventions aimed at bridging the digital divide in healthcare are very important so that people—often the most vulnerable and likely to benefit, are not left behind. Initiatives such as community outreach, digital literacy programs, and user-centred design principles are all strategies to empower patients and enhance their digital health literacy.

Questions Relating to Digital Inclusion in Healthcare Delivery

Today, digital exclusion can be seen as a form of inequality. There is a close correlation between digital exclusion and social disadvantages including lower income, lower levels of education, and poor housing (see Fig. 12.1 below). Medical services working through technological routes need to be accessible and at the planning and review stages need to ask a variety of relevant questions.

Digital Skills   Being able to use the internet and digital devices are critical. Are there programmes in place to equitably extend digital literacy? Do these programmes support good mental health, digital citizenship and safe digital engagement?

Digital Divides   Are there demographic and regional inequalities with respect to digital engagement? Has this been assessed? Do these overlap with healthcare inequalities and social determinants of health? Whose digital rights are most at risk? Do these overlap with people whose 'right to health' may be risk?

Patients and Communities Have local communities been inclusively consulted on the impact of new digital health technologies? Are there (non-digital) patient and user feedback mechanisms to support product improvement?

Connectivity Does the target population have access to the internet with sufficient coverage, through broadband, wi-fi and mobile, but also a consistent power supply? People need the right infrastructure, but this is only the start.

Availability and Accessibility Services must designed to meet all users' needs, including those dependent on assistive technology to access digital services.

Accountability Are all technology suppliers held to account, and challenged to ensure their products are digitally inclusive? Does patient safety, confidentiality and wellbeing remain a priority at each stage of design and deployment?

And more broadly,

Service Commissioners/Providers Are there inclusive initiatives in place to ensure service providers have the digital literacy and skills required to use digital health technology efficiently and securely? Are providers trained to ensure vulnerable populations are not further marginalised by digital health tools?

Digital Policies, Strategies & Compliance Is there a full suite of national digital policies and strategies, and are there systems for implementation compliance? Do these policies/strategies specifically target excluded groups? Do these groups overlap with those who have particular healthcare needs?

Digital solutions may be seen as cheaper and easier to implement but this is problematic when there is failure to consult, review and include all members of the target population. It will take concerted effort to ensure the push for digital ways of working can help tackle health inequalities rather than exacerbate them. Supporting people to get online and use digital health resources can be crucial to achieving local

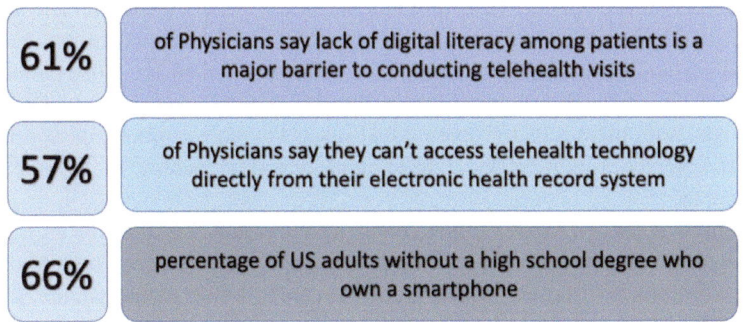

Fig. 12.1 Smartphone and tech usage statistics. Source: COVID-19 Healthcare Coalition and Pew Research Centre [6]

priorities including physical and mental wellbeing; prevention; self-care; shared care and shared decision making; long term condition management; and the appropriate use of urgent and emergency care.

The implications of digital exclusion in healthcare include the health information divide (certain groups will suffer from reduced access to important healthcare information—what services can I access, how do I manage my conditions, who do I contact when things go wrong etc). There will also be missed opportunities for preventative care and early diagnosis. There will be challenges in medication management if people are not able to get in contact with health services easily or understand issues relating to side effects. Additionally digital exclusion may give rise to strained patient-provider relationships if people cannot get in contact with their relevant healthcare professionals to discuss their problems. This leads to ethical problems relating to digital inequity and the potential for harm due to relatively diminished health service provision for excluded groups, whilst the sharp-elbowed middle classes can take full advantage of the suite of digital options available.

Is It Possible to Fix the Fundamentals of Digital Exclusion?

The provision of internet enabled devices is one approach, local authorities or health services could purchase or loan these on behalf of the patient groups that would benefit from them the most—almost as a form of therapeutic intervention in their own right, given that we know that internet access provides both general and specific benefits including empowerment, autonomy and improved quality of life. Alternatively, these could be funded via third sector organisations, sponsorship by local or national businesses or through partnership with the tech industry (although one would have to be mindful of data governance). In Stoke on Trent in the UK, the adult social care team provided elderly clients living in deprived circumstances a smart speaker with a screen to introduce them to a simple technology tool and provide them with a digital assistant [7]. The outcomes of this intervention included positive impacts on people reporting that they were better able to manage their own health conditions and lead more independent lives. The report authors also mentioned that an unexpected outcome of the project was that, for those patients who live alone or are solitary for most of the day having something to talk to that responds, tells them a fact or even a bad joke, was very comforting, and it seems that the device can provide a potentially welcome source of companionship for people.

Another approach for those that already have internet enabled devices, is the supply of data credit. If one is reliant on internet services through a mobile data network, reaching the end of your data allowance can be very problematic. Charities such as National Data Bank and SimPal provide people in need with data in order to support their needs and overcome this access barrier to digital services. There also needs to consideration of affordable provision of home broadband for those people who are less well-off and have dependent health requirements.

Skills development and confidence building are important for the tech naïve. Local libraries, charities and community organisations have developed courses and one to one training initiatives especially aimed at the previously digitally excluded members of society that are delivered by volunteers. Medical services training might relate to how to identify and access local services such as pharmacies and how to use mHealth programmes. Many local health services have now created online video content to guide and explain services to patients and this can be more accessible than written information.

As well as facilitating access to digital services, healthcare providers need to be thoughtful about how they are delivered. Feedback is therefore essential to make sure they are matching their digital solutions and new pathways of care with the goals and capabilities of their target population. Simply asking about communication preferences is an important approach rather than just assuming that everyone wants to be emailed. If a healthcare provider wishes to develop a digitally supported service, then it should build in varying levels of digital interaction so that it can cater to the requirements of the spectrum of patients from the tech savvy to the digitally naïve who still want to rely on physical correspondence and telephone calls.

Levels of Tech Interaction for Healthcare Services
No-tech option—uses letters, phone calls and face to face consultations
   Low-tech intervention—combination of digital access with support from other members of the community
   High-tech option—digital first interaction through online websites and Apps.

Co-creating digital solutions—several different approaches have been found to reduce digital exclusion by improving accessibility. The Mum and Baby App, for example, was developed by the maternity team at the Chelsea and Westminster Hospital in Northwest London. It is a personal guide for pregnancy and labour and was designed by expectant mothers, midwives, and Doctors in order to provide women with all of the relevant information that they need during the maternity period. This couldn't have been successful without close collaboration. Leila Melham, from Hillingdon said *"I really like the app, it feels very comforting. I never knew there was so much to know. Being able to note my thoughts, questions and feelings means it's easier to remember things I want to discuss with my midwife"* [8].

Digital exclusion can only be dealt with through a concerted and holistic approach to overcoming the underlying exacerbating factors. Services have to meet patient needs and be developed with them rather than imposed. Healthcare providers need to become advocates for digitally excluded patients. Working with stakeholders and providing access to equipment, training and encouragement are important to help

Table 12.2 Approaches to improving digital inclusion

Amplifying digital inclusion	
Assessing the status of digital health	Tackling digital exclusion
Understanding local joint strategic needs	Community engagement and public awareness campaigns
Local digital maturity assessment—insights into the local digital environment, infrastructure and policies	Digital inclusion gap analysis based on local and national standards
Understanding local digital transformation plans and capabilities (of both the healthcare workforce but also end users) and digital literacy	Change management plans to improve digital literacy for staff and workforce
Assessing training needs and education plans of healthcare professionals	Procurement frameworks that require digital inclusion assessment

support the increased uptake of digital technologies and online services, as well as working to build trust when bridging gaps. If this approach is not taken, then inequalities will widen between the digital haves and have nots.

At a policy and strategic level, there needs to be consistent guidance about ensuring that digital exclusion is addressed and that there are regulatory frameworks that healthcare providers need to comply with. Countries leading the way in terms of digital healthcare inclusion include Portugal, Denmark, Estonia, Sweden and Finland, all of which have made concerted efforts to upskill their healthcare workers and engage the general population [9]. These countries are able to push the digital health agenda by consistently using the same approaches for data and digital tools across all public services, as well as developing a clear and transparent way of using digital services in order to foster confidence and trust. This is supported by good governance and ensuring that all stakeholders are consulted in a meaningful way (see Table 12.2 below).

Local health systems can support digital inclusion through both high level executive sponsorship and consistency of messaging about the advantages of digital health, grass roots support through the development and encouragement of digital champions, digital skills training across the board, identification of the most at risk and most in need patients in the population, and supporting their transition to digital (for example providing internet connectivity in care homes), mandating and enforcing interoperability standards so that new and old technologies can speak to each other, and providing clear care navigation for digital users so that people can be supported to use health and care services in an optimal way. Co-design of healthcare innovations represents an opportunity to leverage the knowledge, experiences, and insights of end-users to achieve more impactful innovations in real world contexts.

The benefits of assertively and optimistically promoting digital inclusion are multiple and include the increased take up of digital health tools and services; more appropriate use of services including primary and urgent care; reduced pressure on frontline services; time, cost and efficiency savings; better patient activation, medication adherence and treatment compliance, amongst others. There is no guarantee however that such positive benefits can be realised until digital solutions are inclusive and meet the expectations of service users and healthcare professionals.

References

1. NHS England. What we mean by digital inclusion. https://digital.nhs.uk/about-nhs-digital/corporate-information-and-documents/digital-inclusion/what-digital-inclusion-is
2. Lloyds Bank. UK consumer digital index 2022. https://www.lloydsbank.com/assets/media/pdfs/banking_with_us/whats-happening/221103-lloyds-consumer-digital-index-2022-report.pdf
3. Hinton D, Kumar A, Levin B, et al. Are states ready to close the US digital divide? 2022. https://www.mckinsey.com/industries/public-sector/our-insights/are-states-ready-to-close-the-us-digital-divide
4. Spanakis P, Peckham E, Mathers A, Shiers D, Gilbody S. The digital divide: amplifying health inequalities for people with severe mental illness in the time of COVID-19. Br J Psychiatry. 2021;219(4):529–31. https://doi.org/10.1192/bjp.2021.56.
5. World Economic Forum. The global risks report 2021. https://www.weforum.org/publications/the-global-risks-report-2021/
6. Modern Healthcare. Data points: for telehealth to thrive, digital divide needs to close. https://www.modernhealthcare.com/technology/data-points-telehealth-thrive-digital-divide-needs-close
7. Chambers R, Beaney P. The potential of placing a digital assistant in patients' homes. Br J Gen Pract. 2020;70(690):8–9. https://doi.org/10.3399/bjgp20X707273.
8. Bird M, McGillion M, Chambers EM, et al. A generative co-design framework for healthcare innovation: development and application of an end-user engagement framework. Res Involv Engagem. 2021;7:12. https://doi.org/10.1186/s40900-021-00252-7.
9. The Nuffield Trust. What can we learn about digital health care from other countries? https://www.nuffieldtrust.org.uk/news-item/what-can-we-learn-about-digital-health-care-from-other-countries#:~:text=Our%20report%20published%20today%20looks,progress%20on%20digital%20health%20care

Further Reading

Good Things Foundation. Building a digital nation. https://www.goodthingsfoundation.org/insights/building-a-digital-nation/
The Kings Fund. Moving from exclusion to inclusion in digital health and care, 2023. https://www.kingsfund.org.uk/publications/exclusion-inclusion-digital-health-care#:~:text=Groups%20commonly%20considered%20digitally%20excluded,areas%2C%20people%20from%20low%20socio%2D

Chapter 13
The Governance and Ethics of Medical Innovation

Abstract Medical innovation in the digital age has ushered in a transformative era of healthcare, where cutting-edge technologies and digital health solutions hold the promise of improving patient outcomes, enhancing clinical practice, and reducing healthcare costs. However, with great innovation comes the responsibility of addressing the complex issues surrounding governance and ethics. In this chapter, we will explore the complex nature of these challenges, offering insights into the critical considerations that must underpin the development and deployment of new technologies. Importantly we must recognise the importance of not losing the humanity and caring nature of what we are trying to achieve amidst the rush to innovate and dream big.

Keywords Clinical governance · Medical ethics · Moral decisions · Innovation · Digital health revolution · Data privacy and security · Autonomy · Beneficence · Justice · Non-maleficence · Doctor–patient relationship

What's the Problem?

Digital innovation is transforming health care—it is improving service delivery and health outcomes for many people and communities around the world. New technologies are already improving the accuracy, efficiency, and accessibility of medical care. However, fast-moving developments, software evolution, new devices and systems are often created and implemented before strong governance, or the right legislation is in place to ensure safety and privacy. Policies and ethical considerations can take a while to catch up, and the law often follows medicine.

There is a famous line in the film Jurassic Park, in which Jeff Goldblum's character, Dr. Ian Malcolm, states that the scientists were so pre-occupied with whether or not they could make a scientific advance, that they didn't stop to think if they should. This gets to the heart of the ethical concern with all technology. Despite concerted efforts to establish appropriate governance and regulation for digital health, the speed of innovation often outpaces their development and roll out. Laws and guidelines are now needed to cover previously inconceivable advances in medicine. The Canadian province of British Columbia, for example, became the first legislature in the world to expand the potential numbers of parents on a birth certificate to include up to four named individuals, given the developments in artificial reproductive technologies and the use of mitochondrial DNA, meaning that newborn babies can have multiple biological parents, something previously unconceivable (and very difficult to legislate for) [1].

As the digital health revolution continues to promise transformational advancements in healthcare, it is crucial that we also acknowledge our collective responsibility to address potential unintended consequences. Biased and opaque medical algorithms for example have the potential to worsen health disparities and undermine public trust, making it imperative for us to take proactive measures.

An interesting example of how things might go wrong involves data protection and consent. When the Royal Free Hospital in North London decided to work with Google Deepmind the goal was to help develop an innovative software solution for the identification of patients with deteriorating renal function (so called acute kidney injury) during hospital admission. The application called Streams was being designed to develop predictive healthcare alerts and notify clinicians when a patient's biochemistry results were worsening. Acute kidney injury is linked to approximately 40,000 patient deaths per year [2].

However, it was found by the Information Commissioner's Office (the UK's data protection watchdog) that the Hospital (who were the designated data controller) failed to comply with the Data Protection Act when it handed over the data of more than one and a half million people to Deepmind [3]. Service users had not been informed that their personal medical data would be shared with a third party for the purposes of testing an app, it therefore did not have a valid legal basis for the use of the data. The Information Commissioner said, *"Patients would not have reasonably expected their information to have been used in this way, and the Trust could and should have been far more transparent with patients as to what was happening"* [3].

Google responded by saying, *"we underestimated the complexity of the NHS and of the rules around patient data, as well as the potential fears about a well-known tech company working in health. We got that wrong, and we need to do better"* [4].

Therefore, the convergence of new, rapidly advancing technologies in the health sector presents a multitude of ethical, legal and governance challenges. These arise from various factors, including the involvement of new stakeholders such as technology giants, digital therapeutic start-ups and citizen scientists, the vast amounts of data being generated, the use of novel computational and analytic techniques, the excitement and momentum behind new technologies and a lack of regulatory controls or universal standards at present to guide this convergence. Addressing these challenges requires a professional approach that carefully considers the implications for all stakeholders involved in the ever-evolving digital health ecosystem.

Perspectives on Digital Health

The general public, patients and policy makers are generally positive about the promise of digital health technologies. It's seen as a way of advancing medical care with the added benefits of convenience, accessibility and (hopefully) cost-effectiveness. There is overall an optimistic and positive understanding of the role of digital health interventions. A competing perspective for those in the health sector however, is that the widespread adoption of digital technologies in healthcare will increasingly raise ethical issues, impacting on domains of self, identity, social acceptability, personal autonomy, equality, responsibility and justice. So far it has generally been the case that any ethical problems are confined to the features of the device or technology itself, such as privacy, security, data governance, consent, etc. These are often discussed in terms of the fundamental concepts of beneficence and non-maleficence, respect for autonomy and equality of access (justice) [5]. Shaw and Donia, researchers from the Institute of Health Policy, Management and Evaluation in Toronto, writing in Frontiers in Digital Health, criticise this narrow, principalist view and argue that this is disconnected from the broader impact and implications of the adoption of digital health products on the wider health care system and the society that it is part of, (for example transparency, accountability and fairness), and a much broader analysis is required to inform the distribution of benefits and burdens that emanate from the use of new health tech [6].

The main areas in which this broader view is apparent include the influence of large technology companies over public health policy and their access to large swathes of personal health data, the fact that health technologies will have a significant impact on the way we live our lives and the way we interact with health services—and how those health services are designed and delivered, the potential inequalities between groups and populations (the haves and the have nots) and the variance in impact that technologies might have based on proximity. Those close to a technology, may be affected by trust and privacy issues for example, whilst those further away suffer from lack of resources or ability to implement new technologies. Challenges such as privacy and security might be framed as technical challenges and it is in the interests of technology developers and digital health advocates to keep attention focused on the technical aspects and fixes, rather than on more substantial moral and ethical implications.

Main Challenges Facing Digital Health

Patient Autonomy Over Data Usage Issues over data access, data sharing and data security are hot topics in the field of digital health alongside the freedoms of informed consent and choice. Often patients find that their medical data is automatically shared or collated by other providers under presumed consent or active opt-out scenarios and feel aggrieved that they never had an awareness or opportunity to understand more about what is involved. From the individual's perspective it does not always feel that information is private or secure. Decisions appear to have been taken on their behalf by a higher authority (for reasons of convenience) and valid informed consent should be actively taken considering long-term data storage and use.

Governance of Healthcare Data Safe, transparent and appropriate use of medical data is critical. The majority of patients would expect that their records to be kept private and confidential and that only people involved in their care would have access to it. Data needs to be stored in such a way that it is protected from unauthorised access and data breaches, as well as not being sold on to third parties for commercial reasons.

Responsible Use of Data and Technologies by Healthcare Professionals The responsible use of data and digital health solutions are imperative as we proceed into a more digitised medical future. It is possible that the busy clinician may use ChatGPT to develop a management plan for a patient, only to find out later that the information generated was incorrect but also biased and replete with risks (because the underlying algorithms informing the treatment strategy were based on a cohort of North American middle aged Caucasian males). Similarly with clinical decision support systems it is important that the clinician remains accountable and does not outsource their professional responsibilities or thought processes to a rules based or AI influenced approach that does not take specific individual patient characteristics into consideration. A comparison with autonomously driving vehicles is relevant here as we are still not at the stage yet where these cars are allowed to be completely driverless—someone still needs to have their hands on the steering wheel both literally and figuratively. There is a potential for trust in the Doctor-patient relationship to be damaged if individuals think that their healthcare provider is just letting a machine do all the work and failing to see them as an individual.

Equity in Digital Health As mentioned in earlier chapters, the risk of a widening digital divide is clear. Individual equity and inclusion in the field of digital health relates to empowerment, accessibility and getting fair treatment. Those who are digitally excluded may potentially be stigmatised, discriminated against and left behind because they are not empowered and unable to access the benefits of new technologies and this digital poverty further compounds the underlying social determinants of poor health.

Examples of what Shaw and Donia describe as a 'sociotechnical' approach to digital health ethics include the negative mental health consequences of being constantly tracked and surveyed through remote health technologies [6]. This may manifest as the fear of not achieving perfection, feelings of being a failure, letting the Doctor down and being worried about what others will think of you. This is already apparent in the field of diabetes care where patients use implanted continuous glucose monitoring to record their ambulatory glucose profiles all day, every day and the results are shared via the cloud to their local diabetes team who can review and comment on their food intake and activities (see Figs. 13.1 and 13.2 below).

Prior to such technologies, people would only measure their finger prick blood glucose results 3 or 4 times a day and either store their results on a hand-held glucometer or write them down in a little booklet so that one could learn how and when to adjust one's insulin does. If an erroneous blood glucose result arose, due to '*being naughty*'—'*Sorry Doctor it was my birthday*' then it could either be omitted from the records or hidden completely (truck drivers with Diabetes for example need to legally keep a fastidious record of their blood glucose values before and during driving and present their glucose meter—which has a 90 day memory—for review on a regular basis. One classic way round this was to have two glucose meters, one to capture all the results and one to use for the best results to show the Diabetologist). This is no longer possible with continuous monitoring and can potentially precipitate anxiety, distress and non-engagement amongst patients. The power of digital health technologies to influence mental well-being should not be underestimated.

Several forms of digital health applications that use algorithms (for example clinical decision support tools) run the risk of causing both ethical and practical harms, because of the foundational elements that comprise the rule set that goes into them [7]. Much of health technology (like a great deal of pharmacology) is based on the needs of a standardised population of certain groups whose characteristics are not relevant to large numbers of other people in our society. This means that for individuals and marginalised groups outside of this presumed mainstream, there is the risk of bias, less accuracy, and anomalous outcomes for those who don't conform to the stereotypical end-user. Additionally, algorithms can have the appearance of a black box because we cannot see the components of decision-making outputs, which may be based on structural inaccuracies and assumptions.

Impact on the Doctor–Patient Relationship

The interaction between a shaman or healer, a village elder, a Doctor, and the recipient of particular treatment, has long been held as sacred and a powerful catalyst to the healing process. 'The Doctor as a drug' significantly enhances the placebo effect ('I shall please') and the way that clinicians relate to their patients, their bedside manner, their time, patience, and attention is well recognised to influence how people respond and adhere to their treatments. Whilst online and remote, or automated medical care processes are rapidly expanding (and convenient and cheaper), it will be interesting to observe how the outcomes of traditional in-person care, compare to the digitally mediated forms of healthcare delivery, on both a qualitative and quantitative level. This is a hot ethical topic, as removing the Doctor, by increments, from care delivery, is an ethical issue, both potentially harmful and potentially liberating. Certainly, it could also be seen as a way of democratising healthcare

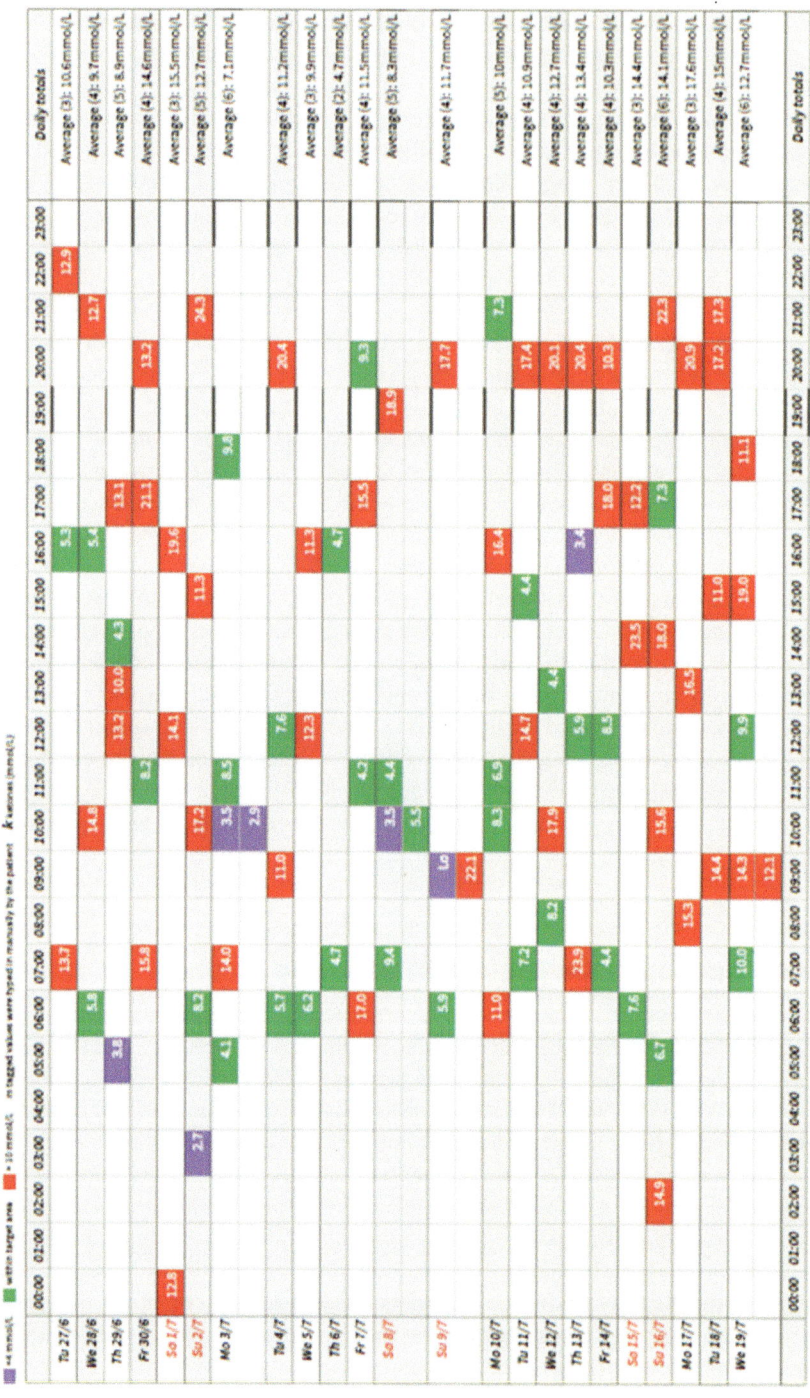

Fig. 13.1 Glucose monitor results download. Normal range results are in green, low readings are in purple and those readings that are high/above range are in stigmatising red

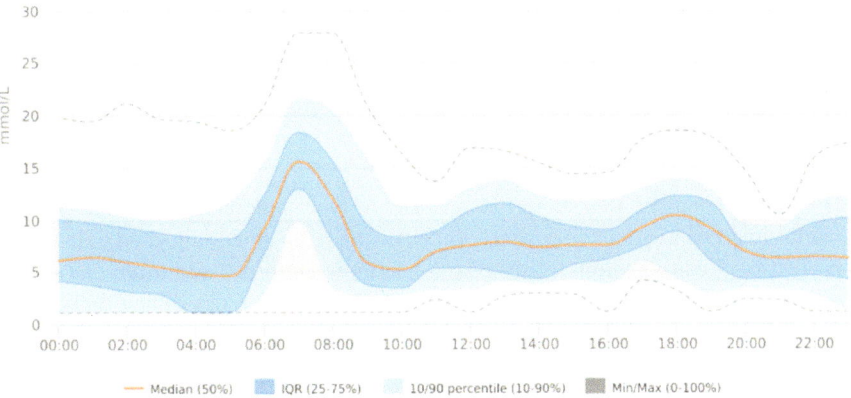

Fig. 13.2 Ambulatory Glucose Profile (AGP) based on continuous glucose monitoring device outputs

and empowering patients by removing the esteemed Doctor as a facilitator of healthcare delivery (and their paternalistic and biased behaviour and the risk of malpractice) and moving things towards a self-service model of care delivery. After all what is a Doctor, but a combination of a highly trained pattern recognition machine combined with a beneficent and charming prescription provider? It's this second element that offers the most food for thought. The diagnostic, recipe driven investigation protocol can be replicated by machine learning (based on 1000's of Doctors experience) but the friendly, kind and endearing, hand-holding relationship is one that cannot be reproduced, and this is the most significant potential detriment of digitally mediated care. For many conditions, conveyor belt transactional care is actually fine. Something is broken and I need to get it fixed. However, the human impact of disease is more profound and complex and can't easily be simulated or left out, for many conditions, and it is this factor that we need to ensure that we do not forget as we move forwards into the brave new world of tech.

Impact on the Doctor

The increased utilisation of digital health systems and processes generally involves adapting long established and traditional processes or routines and this can raise multiple ethical and legal dilemmas. An interesting study by Anna Silven from the Department of Public Health and Primary Care in the Netherlands looked into the views of various stakeholders in order to identify challenges regarding responsibility and liability when using digital health in clinical practice [8]. This was part of an overarching project aiming to explore the most pressing ethical and legal obstacles regarding the implementation and adoption of digital health in the Netherlands, and to propose actionable solutions. The emerging general theme was '*uncertainty regarding responsibilities*' when adopting digital health solutions. Key dilemmas appear to take place in clinical settings and within the doctor-patient relationship. Although legal frameworks governing medical practice describe core ethical principles, rights and obligations of physicians, they do not always suffice to clearly clarify their responsibilities in the setting of digital health. In the absence of appropriate legal guidance and codes of conduct tailored specifically to this new field, Doctors' responsibilities should relate back to their general duty of care. In other words, to do what is best for patients (not causing harm and doing good). Healthcare professional organisations could take a leading role to provide more clarity with respect to Doctors' responsibility, by developing guidance describing their duty of care in the context of digital, and to address their new resulting responsibilities. Silven's team made the following recommendations about professional responsibilities to help overcome this issue;

- Professional/medical associations should play an active role in supporting physicians in the adoption of digital health.
- When possible, Doctors should act and prescribe based on the organisational endorsement of evidence-based digital health, by for example, a healthcare institution or a professional association.
- Doctors should actively contribute to the establishment of evidence-based digital health.
- A new part of the Doctors job is to carry out a holistic evaluation of the patient which includes (digital) health literacy.
- When providing a digital health intervention, communicate about the intended use in order to align patients' expectations to the intended benefits.
- Communicate about patients' responsibilities and explain the risks of adopting digital health.
- Communicate about the steps to discontinue the use of digital health and offer alternative treatment options.

Data Inference

'Human Resources' is an awful way of describing and dehumanising an organisation's workforce. Considering them to be units of productivity or cogs in a machine is not uncommon. Occupational health departments exist in large companies and public sector organisations in order to keep the workers active and at work. There are many potential opportunities for digital health and monitoring technologies to track and analyse human behaviours, collect data and make inferences about an individual's utility (and usefulness). This becomes relevant when health insurance gets in on the act, assessing which humans are highly productive and low risk, and those who have high risk characteristics. The classic example here comes from blood pressure measurement. In the early twentieth century when blood pressure monitoring was seen as a novelty, it was insurance companies who crunched the numbers and saw the correlation between blood pressure trends and morbidity and mortality. They were then able to categorise people into different risk bands and set their premiums accordingly. We do not yet know what insights may be gleaned about our health and prognostic outlook based on our digital data, but it will become an increasingly thorny ethical issue to see people reduced to a numerical risk score based on the data collected on them through their smartwatch, smart toilet and snippets of conversation captured by their smart speakers.

Digital Rights Surrounding Access Inequality

We've already mentioned the problems with disparate digital infrastructure across countries (remote and rural areas) and across the world. Lack or absence of adequate broadband and Wi-Fi for digital health technologies to work on will continue to be a big problem for many years to come and exacerbates the divide between the digital haves and have nots. Corporations which install infrastructure may not see it as economically worthwhile to offer connection to harder to reach communities.

The concept of internet access as a fundamental right, also referred to as broadband freedom or the freedom to connect, asserts that every individual should have the ability to use the internet in order to exercise and fully experience their rights to free expression, opinion, and other essential human rights [9]. It is arguably the duty of governments to guarantee that internet access is widely accessible and not unjustly blocked for any individual.

Material and Device Supply Chains

It is hard to argue against the importance of having internet access, many of us would struggle to live our lives without it. However, we need to balance this need with the negative environmental impacts of the technologies that we have come to rely on so much. We are all in part responsible for damage to ecosystems, complicity with corrupt regimes and human rights abuses by possessing a smart phone for example, because of the materials contained within, mined from a facility deep within Africa, worked by low paid workers, guarded by child soldiers and propped up by unpleasant governments. But because this is far away and we can't see it, it is easy to ignore and shift our focus. This benefits both us and large technology corporations who feast on high levels of digital consumption in developed nations. This creates an ethical tension in digital health—should we use such technologies because of the unethical way in which they are sourced, or discount such worries because of the greater good?

Government Policy and Regulation

The ways in which we decide how societies use new technologies, will not be decided by me or you, they will be influenced by the powerful lobbyists, consultants and corporate actors who seek to benefit most from the increased uptake of digital health, the licensing of software, the selling and marketing of our personal health information and the targeted raising of insurance premiums. This is because the regulatory and legal agenda has shifted from democratic control into the hands of those who have most to profit from the manipulation of healthcare systems strategy and operations and their shareholders. Huge numbers of private companies are following the gold-rush into the digital health market, (not all for beneficent reasons). This is perhaps the biggest ethical dilemma of all, that digital health will be marketed as a panacea for all ills, conducive to profit generation, but not necessarily patients' best interests. This is why a balanced ethical approach not just along principalist lines, but also to take into consideration the wider societal implications, needs to be taken and a clear framework for governance of innovation needs to be agreed upon. This may well include using a broad range of perspectives drawn from wider society to provide input into the meaning, acceptability, and desirability of new technologies, as well as exploring the potential negative consequences for various stakeholders. In this new field, the ethics of digital health implementation will matter greatly, because of the increasingly eminent and important role that it will play.

Ways to Overcome Potential Harms of Digital Health

Understanding the current state of digital health governance is key for developing meaningful change in healthcare. There has been significant progress in digital health governance over the last 5 years as stakeholders have worked to rapidly develop and implement new policies and programs to cover a range of governance areas from the efficacy of digital health tools to market access and approvals. All of these, however, attempt to ensure that digital health systems can appropriately respond to health system needs and priorities with transparency and accountability.

Global guidance can help inform better country-level digital health governance. For example, the *Principles for Digital Development* is a community-driven set of living guidance to help digital development practitioners successfully and appropriately apply digital technology in development programs (Box 13.1 below) [10]. Over time, the principles may change as they are updated and modified to fit specific contexts and environments.

Box 13.1 Digital development principles

Principles for Digital Development
- **Design with the user**—understanding of user characteristics, needs and challenges.
- **Understanding the existing ecosystem**—dedicating time and resources to analyse the ecosystem or context helps to ensure that selected technology tools will be relevant and will not duplicate existing efforts.
- **Design for scale**—thinking beyond the pilot and making choices that will enable widespread adoption later.
- **Build for sustainability**—a program built for sustainability is more likely to be embedded into policies, daily practices and user workflow.
- **Be Data Driven**—when an initiative is data driven, quality information is available to the right people when they need it, and they are using that data to take action.
- **Use Open Standards, Open Data, Open Source and Open Innovation**—an open approach to digital development can help to increase collaboration in the digital development community and avoid duplicating work that has already been done.
- **Reuse and improve**—look for ways to adapt and enhance existing products, resources and approaches.
- **Address privacy and security**—careful consideration of which data are collected and how data are acquired, used, stored and shared.
- **Be Collaborative**—sharing information, insights, strategies and resources across projects, organisations and sectors, leading to increased efficiency and impact.

Similarly, there are a set of Global Health Data Governance Principles which act as a useful resource for policymakers, advocates, and other stakeholders who are working toward equitable, human rights–based approaches to health data governance (Fig. 13.3 below) [11]. They bring a human rights and equity lens to the use all types of data across healthcare systems and are divided into three main categories (protecting people, prioritising equity and promoting health value).

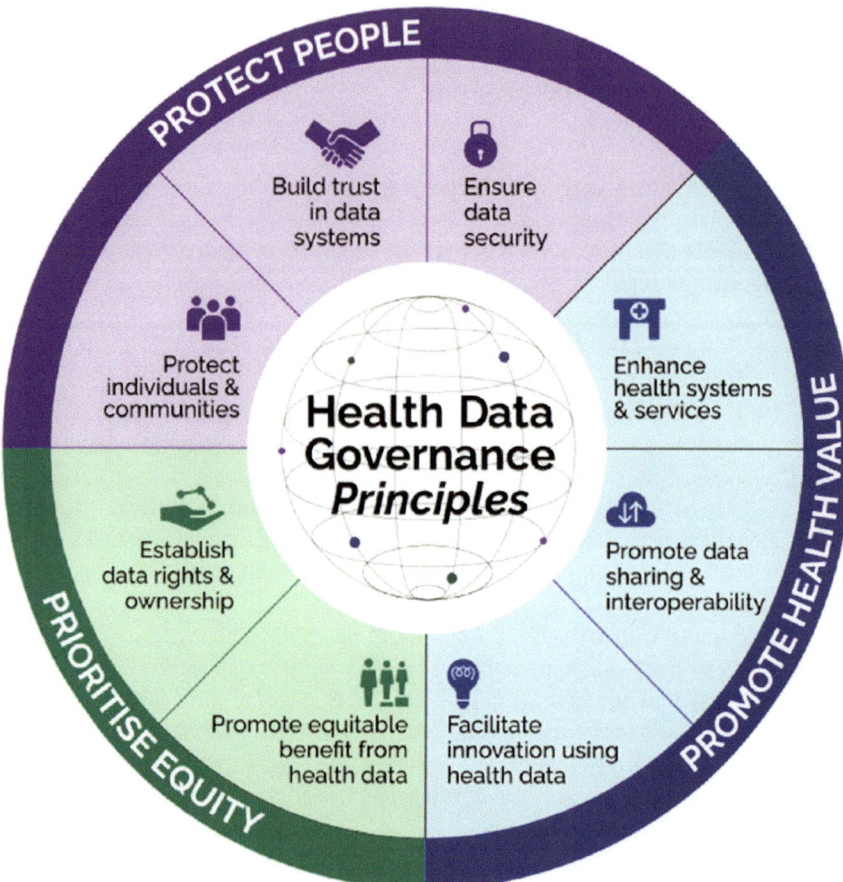

Fig. 13.3 Digital health principles. Reproduced from Holly et al. (2023) [11]. Source: Holly et al. (2023) [11]. https://www.emerald.com/insight/content/doi/10.1108/IJHG-11-2022-0104/full/html under Creative Commons Licence BY 4.0. https://creativecommons.org/licenses/by/4.0/

Governance of Digital Innovation—Doing the Right Things Right

The governance of innovation refers to the framework, policies, rules, and practices that guide and oversee the process of introducing, managing, and regulating innovation within an organisation, industry, or society at large. It involves setting the rules, norms, and mechanisms that ensure innovations are developed, deployed, and maintained in a responsible, effective, and ethical manner.

A recent report by the Institute of Development Studies looking at the rapid growth of digital health services since the emergence of COVID-19 warns that systems of governance have not been able to keep up with the pace of change [12]. This could lead to potentially negative impacts on clinical safety, cost effectiveness, digital equity and access. During the pandemic many authorities rolled back the regulatory constraints around the use of digital health technologies so that healthcare providers and tech companies could more quickly set up digital services. This relaxation of regulation is concerning and there needs to be a universal approach to protecting patients, especially the most vulnerable and marginalised.

The key foundational elements that describe good governance are;

1. **Regulatory Frameworks:** laws and regulations that define what is allowed and what isn't in terms of innovation. Regulatory bodies need to oversee specific digital health technologies to ensure safety, fairness, and compliance with ethical standards.

2. **Ethical Guidelines:** innovation governance often involves a set of ethical principles and guidelines that help innovators make responsible decisions. This can include considerations related to fairness, privacy, transparency, and respect for human rights.

3. **Standards and Best Practices:** many industries establish standards and best practices to ensure the quality and safety of innovations. These can be set by industry associations or international bodies; however self-regulation can often have flaws and be seen as unenforceable.

4. **Intellectual Property Rights:** rules and laws around patents, copyrights, trademarks, and other forms of intellectual property protection encourage innovation by ensuring inventors can benefit from their work. However, this needs to be balanced with the greater good of wider society, a classic example from medical history is that of the eighteenth century Obstetricians who kept the invention of forceps for use in difficult deliveries secret for many years to ensure their own monopoly and profit, whilst many women and babies were lost in childbirth due to being unable to access such a useful and life-saving tool.

5. **Funding and Investment:** policies and practices that guide investment in innovation, including government grants, venture capital, and research funding. Ensuring adequate funding is often a crucial aspect of innovation governance.

6. **Risk Management:** innovation often carries risks, both in terms of safety and viability. Governance involves identifying, assessing, and managing these risks to ensure they are within acceptable limits.

7. **Data Privacy and Security:** with the increasing role of data-driven technologies, there need to be strong rules for protecting the privacy and security of personal data.

8. **Quality Assurance and Testing:** ensuring that innovations meet certain quality and safety standards through testing and validation procedures. This is particularly important in fields like healthcare and aerospace.

9. **Environmental and Social Responsibility:** innovations must also be governed with respect to their environmental and social impact. Sustainability and social responsibility are increasingly important considerations.

10. **Transparency and Accountability:** there should always be transparency in decision-making processes and that those responsible for innovations are held

accountable for their actions (it will be interesting to see how this relates to corporate manslaughter legislation).

11. **Collaboration and Knowledge Sharing:** in many cases, innovation promotes collaboration and knowledge sharing among different stakeholders, including academia, industry, government and other healthcare organisations around the world.

12. **Compliance and Auditing:** monitoring and auditing mechanisms need to be put in place to ensure that organisations and individuals adhere to the established rules and regulations.

In her third report to the Human Rights Council, Tlaleng Mofokeng, UN Special Rapporteur on the right to health, focused on digital technologies and the right to health. She said *"There are a number of global and national efforts that are now underway to strengthen the governance on digital health,"* and added that *"meaningful participation is key"* [13].

Overall, the governance of innovation seeks to strike a balance between encouraging and supporting innovation while also safeguarding against potential risks, ensuring ethical conduct, and fostering responsible and sustainable progress. It plays a critical role in shaping the direction and impact of new technologies and ideas in our rapidly changing world.

The Ethics of Innovation in Digital Health

The ethics of innovation in the field of digital health refers to the moral principles, values, and guidelines that guide the development, deployment, and use of technological advancements and digital solutions within healthcare. Digital health innovations encompass a wide range of technologies, including electronic medical records, telemedicine, wearable devices, health apps, AI, and more. Ethical considerations in this field are essential to ensure that these innovations are designed and implemented in a way that prioritises patient well-being, respects individual rights, and upholds the highest standards of medical ethics.

Beneficence and Non-Maleficence
- The fundamental ethical principles of medical innovation revolve around doing good (beneficence) and avoiding harm (non-maleficence).
- Digital health technologies should be designed to maximise the benefits to patients, whilst minimising potential harms.

Respect for Autonomy
- Patients' autonomy in making informed choices about their health is a cornerstone of medical ethics.

- Digital health tools must respect and support patient autonomy in decision-making, data sharing, and consent.

Justice
- The distribution of healthcare innovations and benefits should be just and equitable, ensuring that new technologies do not exacerbate existing health disparities.
- Accessibility, affordability, and inclusivity are critical factors in the pursuit of fairness in healthcare innovation.

Key elements in delivering the ethics of innovation in digital health include:

1. **Patient-Centred Care:** prioritising the well-being and preferences of patients in the development of digital health solutions is vital. This involves designing tools that empower patients to make informed decisions about their healthcare and ensuring their consent is obtained for data sharing and usage.
2. **Privacy and Data Security:** respecting patient privacy by safeguarding health data and personal information from unauthorised access or breaches. Data should be collected and used with the utmost care, and patients must be informed about how their data will be handled. The increasing reliance on digital systems exposes healthcare to cybersecurity threats. Stringent cybersecurity measures are essential to protect sensitive patient information and the integrity of medical devices.
3. **Informed Consent:** obtaining clear and voluntary consent from patients or users of digital health tools, explaining what data will be collected, how it will be used, and any potential risks or benefits. Developers should ensure that patients have a clear understanding of how their data will be utilised.
4. **Equity and Accessibility:** ensuring that digital health innovations are accessible to all, regardless of socioeconomic status, geography, or physical abilities. Active efforts should be made to bridge the digital divide and reduce healthcare disparities.
5. **Transparency:** providing transparency in the functioning of digital health tools, algorithms, and decision-making processes. Patients and healthcare providers should have a clear understanding of how these technologies work.
6. **Data Ownership and Control:** empowering individuals to have control over their health data, allowing them to access, modify, or share it as they see fit. Patients should be able to opt-out of data sharing if they wish but they must have the right to control their own health data.
7. **Responsibility in AI and Algorithms:** developing and using artificial intelligence and algorithms that are fair, unbiased, and accountable. This involves mitigating bias, ensuring transparency, and monitoring for unintended consequences. Robust training data, diverse data sources, and continuous algorithmic monitoring are essential to overcome problems in this field.

8. **Quality and Efficacy:** ensuring that digital health innovations meet high standards of quality and efficacy. Rigorous testing and validation procedures are crucial to avoid potential harm to patients.
9. **Continual Monitoring and Improvement:** innovators should be committed to ongoing evaluation and improvement of digital health tools based on real-world data and feedback. This is critical for ensuring the effectiveness and safety of these technologies.
10. **Ethical Research and Innovation:** conducting research and innovation in a way that respects the principles of medical ethics and research ethics, including obtaining ethical review board approval for human research and respecting the main ethical principles.
11. **Professional Responsibility:** healthcare providers and professionals must adhere to ethical standards when using digital health tools and must maintain their competence and ethical standards in the use of these technologies.

In summary, the ethics of innovation in digital health centres around the responsible and patient-centric development and use of technology to improve healthcare. This involves balancing the potential benefits of digital health with the ethical responsibilities to protect patient rights, privacy, and safety. It ensures that technology supports, rather than detracts from, the fundamental principles of medical ethics. Both the governance and ethics of medical innovation in the context of new technologies and digital health solutions are of paramount importance as we navigate the rapidly evolving landscape of healthcare. Ethical considerations, regulatory frameworks, data privacy, AI fairness, and patient-centred innovation must all be integrated into the development and deployment of these technologies. Ultimately, a commitment to balancing innovation with ethical responsibility and good governance is essential to ensure the full potential of medical innovation is realised without compromising patient well-being, autonomy, and equity.

Digital health developers must prioritise transparency and evidence of fit, performance, and sustainability for the intended uses of new technologies. Finally, continuous learning and shared experience among health care professionals, ministries of health, and regulatory bodies will ensure a cohesive, holistic approach to the full cycle of development, implementation and evaluation of digital solutions.

References

1. Rolfsen C. Della Wolf is B.C.'s 1st child with 3 parents on birth certificate. 2014. https://www.cbc.ca/news/canada/british-columbia/della-wolf-is-b-c-s-1st-child-with-3-parents-on-birth-certificate-1.2526584
2. Argyropoulos A, Townley S, Upton PM, Dickinson S, Pollard AS. Identifying on admission patients likely to develop acute kidney injury in hospital. BMC Nephrol. 2019;20(1):56. https://doi.org/10.1186/s12882-019-1237-x.
3. Hern A. Royal Free breached UK data law in 1.6m patient deal with Google's DeepMind. https://www.theguardian.com/technology/2017/jul/03/google-deepmind-16m-patient-royal-free-deal-data-protection-act

4. Suleyman M, King D. The Information Commissioner, the Royal Free, and what we've learned. 2017. https://deepmind.google/discover/blog/the-information-commissioner-the-royal-free-and-what-weve-learned/
5. Brall C, Schröder-Bäck P, Maeckelberghe E. Ethical aspects of digital health from a justice point of view. Eur J Pub Health. 2019;29(Supplement_3):18–22.
6. Shaw JA, Donia J. The sociotechnical ethics of digital health: a critique and extension of approaches from bioethics. Front Digit Health. 2021;3:725088. https://doi.org/10.3389/fdgth.2021.725088.
7. Moor JH. Why we need better ethics for emerging technologies. Ethics Inf Technol. 2005;7:111–9. https://doi.org/10.1007/s10676-006-0008-0.
8. Silven AV, van Peet PG, Boers SN, et al. Clarifying responsibility: professional digital health in the doctor-patient relationship, recommendations for physicians based on a multi-stakeholder dialogue in The Netherlands. BMC Health Serv Res. 2022;22:129.
9. Klang M, Murray A. Human rights in the digital age. Routledge; 2005. p. 1.
10. Principles for digital development. https://digitalprinciples.org/
11. Holly L, Thom S, Elzemety M, Murage B, Mathieson K, Iñigo Petralanda MI. Strengthening health data governance: new equity and rights-based principles. Int J Health Gov. 2023;28(3):225–37. https://doi.org/10.1108/IJHG-11-2022-0104.
12. Bloom G, Balasubramaniam P, Marin A, et al. 'Towards digital transformation for universal health coverage'. Mutual learning for mixed health systems. Brighton: Institute of Development Studies; 2023. https://doi.org/10.19088/CC.2023.005.
13. United Nations. UN expert calls for meaningful participation in national and global governance of digital health. 2023. https://www.ohchr.org/en/press-releases/2023/06/un-expert-calls-meaningful-participation-national-and-global-governance

Further Reading

Donia J, Shaw JA. Co-design and ethical artificial intelligence for health: an agenda for critical research and practice. Big Data Soc. 2021;8(2). https://doi.org/10.1177/20539517211065248.
Guston DH. Understanding "anticipatory governance". Soc Stud Sci. 2014;44(2):218–42. https://doi.org/10.1177/0306312713508669.
Nebeker C, Harlow J, Giacinto-Espinoza R, Linares-Orozco R, Bloss C, Weibel N. Ethical and regulatory challenges of research using pervasive sensing and other emerging technologies: IRB perspectives. AJOB Empir Bioeth. 2017;8(4):266–76.
Nebeker C, Torous J, Bartlett Ellis RJ. Building the case for actionable ethics in digital health research supported by artificial intelligence. BMC Med. 2019;17:137. https://doi.org/10.1186/s12916-019-1377-7.
Sharon T. Blind-sided by privacy? Digital contact tracing, the Apple/Google API and big tech's newfound role as global health policy makers. Ethics Inf Technol. 2021;23:45–57. https://doi.org/10.1007/s10676-020-09547-x.
Ummon IJ, Halim KS. The ethical issues in digital healthcare that healthcare professionals should consider - summary of literature review by CiMCH. 2020. https://projects.tuni.fi/digicareasia/digicare-model/the-ethical-issues-in-digital-health-care%E2%80%AFthat-health-care%E2%80%AFprofessionals%E2%80%AFshould%E2%80%AFconsider/
Veinot TC, Mitchell H, Ancker JS. Good intentions are not enough: how informatics interventions can worsen inequality. J Am Med Inform Assoc. 2018;25:1080–8. https://doi.org/10.1093/jamia/ocy052.

Chapter 14
The Future of Hospitals and Digital Health

Abstract The future of digital health holds immense potential to improve patient outcomes, enhance healthcare delivery, and increase the efficiency of healthcare systems. It is likely to be characterised by significant advancements, innovations, and transformative changes in healthcare delivery and our society. However, it also raises important ethical and regulatory questions that need to be addressed to ensure responsible and equitable implementation. Additionally, as the field continues to evolve, stakeholders must remain vigilant in safeguarding patient privacy and data security, and ultimately the humanity of Doctor-patient relationships.

Keywords Future medicine · Future healthcare · Digital health · Ethics of medical innovation · Artifical intelligence · Stem cells · Precision medicine · Digital therapeutics

The Future Healthcare Landscape

The doctor of the future will give no medication but will interest his patients in the care of the human frame, diet and in the cause and prevention of disease—Thomas A. Edison

The drivers of change in health care have long been with us, the rising burden of illness, systemic inequalities, the high costs of healthcare delivery, the desperate need for better prevention and population health and the widening capacity chasm of health services. Technology is seen as a significant enabler in being able to deliver the healthcare of the future, allowing a change in the way that medical care is delivered, how patients interact with services and a shift of medical care down a gradient away from the old Hospital and into homes, communities, and the hands of patients. The ultimate goal being to reduce our societal burden of disease and close the demand-capacity gap that makes it so difficult for us to progress in the here and now [1].

The near future will see the increasing ubiquity of digital health technologies and a growth in their functionalities, to enable a more joined up way of delivering healthcare (Fig. 14.1). A major change will be in the nature of Hospitals themselves. With

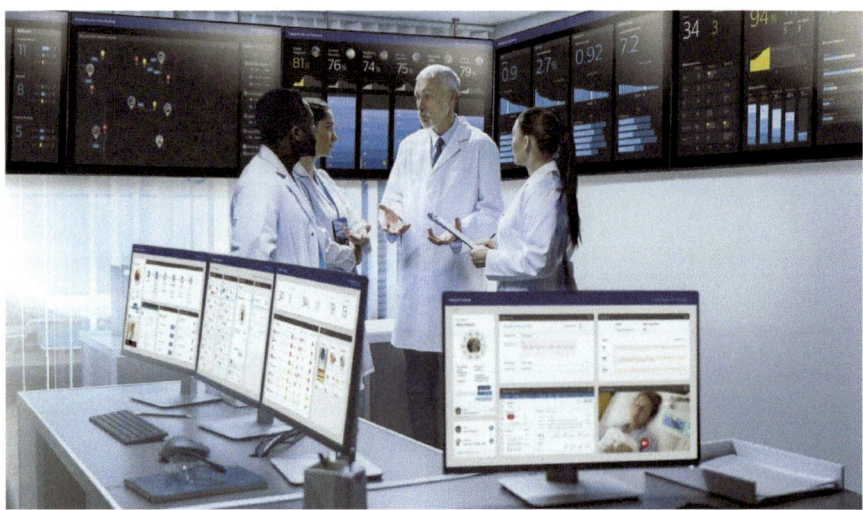

Fig. 14.1 Future doctors. Reproduced with permissions from Philips Media Library (https://www.philips.com/a-w/about/news/media-library.html)

appropriate planning and imagination these will become smaller as there will be less need for both outpatient and in-patient spaces, and emergency demands will be lessened through digital solutions and services such as virtual clinics and targeted prevention for at-risk individuals [2]. The residual Hospital estate will be an intelligent system that looks after the sickest patients who require intensive care and monitoring, tracks operational flow and optimises care delivery, resulting in limited Hospital stays and greater patient safety. There will also hopefully be a much greater focus on patient centric design. Hospitals of the future should prioritise user experience to create environments that promote healing, reduce stress, and enhance the overall patient journey. This could involve more comfortable, calming and adaptable spaces, access to natural light, and the integration of art and nature into hospital design.

With regards to the way that services are designed and delivered we have already seen how remote monitoring and virtual care delivery can improve the patient journey, cut down or eliminate the Hospital visits and speed up the time between referral and definitive treatment. Shifting from the '*we've always done it like this*' mentality will support creative and more patient focussed ways of meeting the needs of patients. At an organisational and system level, a holistic approach will mean that there will be less variation in care, greater quality control and a performance management mechanism for ensuring that the best care is being delivered. There may even be a *nationalisation* of health services in which resources and information are shared and that clinicians work across the wider network to provide care in a distributed manner.

The impact on healthcare professionals will be profound. Hopefully they will be freed from the many arduous barriers and time-consuming administrative processes involved in their daily work, as these become automated, and they will be allowed to focus on clinical decision making and direct patient care, supported by intelligent

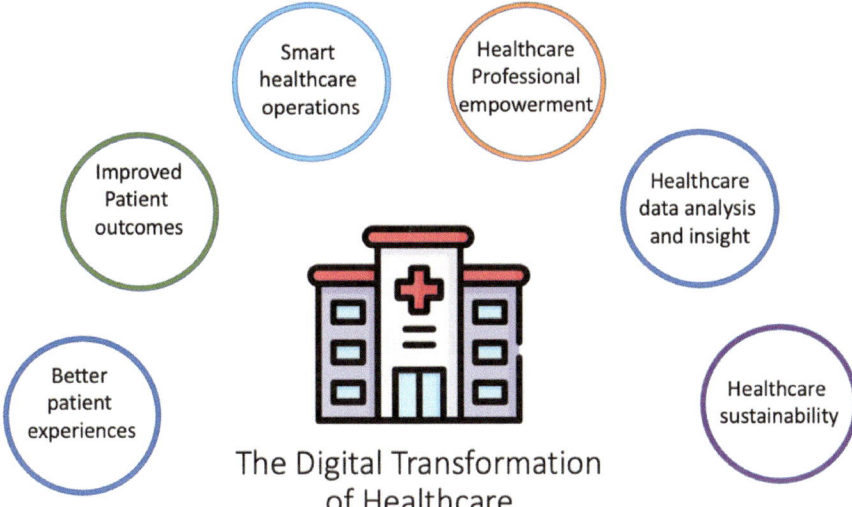

Fig. 14.2 Domains of future healthcare development

systems that can safely compliment their work. Training will be required for the clinician of the future to have the capabilities required to work in a digital healthcare system, but the majority of Doctors and Nurses already recognise and want to take advantage of digital solutions. Technology will allow clinicians to spend more time with their patients and take their eyes off the computer screen (see Fig. 14.2 below).

The impact on patients will be at two extremes of a spectrum. Firstly, greater empowerment through access to medical data and clinicians, transparency about what is happening with their care and greater accessibility and convenience overall, which will lead to greater satisfaction. However, there will also be a widening digital divide in those people and communities who cannot use digital health technologies for whatever reason. This runs the risk of even more unequal care provision and needs to be actively tackled so that lack of technical opportunities does not become another social determinant of health. A major focus of a future healthcare initiatives is to overcome digital exclusion as described in Chap. 12.

Domains of Digital Health

A big push for virtual models of care took place between 2020 and 2022 as a consequence of the global COVID pandemic [3]. The challenges presented by lockdown were addressed through a widespread adoption of remote care, utilising straightforward solutions. A notable instance was the implementation of virtual early discharge respiratory wards, where patients received follow-up via telephone or video communication with a medical professional. In addition, they were provided with an oxygen saturation monitor and given instructions on whom to contact in case of clinical decline. This approach proved to be both safe and well-received by patients, while also being cost-efficient in delivering quality care within the home setting.

The following categories summarise the areas in which technological systems and new digital services will bring about clinical-digital transformation.

Widespread Adoption of Telemedicine This gained significant momentum during the pandemic and is likely to become a permanent fixture in healthcare. It will continue to evolve with improved video and remote monitoring technologies, expanding access to care and reducing the burden on healthcare facilities.

Artificial Intelligence and Machine Learning AI will play a central role in digital health. These technologies will be used for predictive analytics, pattern recognition, early disease detection, personalised treatment plans, and more. AI-powered virtual assistants will become more prevalent in healthcare settings.

Remote Monitoring The use of wearable devices and IoT sensors for continuous patient monitoring will grow. This will enable healthcare providers to collect real-time data on patients' health, improving the management of chronic conditions and enhancing preventive care. There will be an increase in the use of home diagnostics and early alert systems, many of which will be built into the fabric of our homes (and toilets).

Precision Medicine Advances in genomics, proteomics, and data analytics will drive the growth of precision medicine. Tailoring medical treatment (pharmacogenomics) and interventions to an individual's genetic makeup and health profile will become increasingly common.

Prescription Digital Therapeutics This involves the use of software guidance to treat specific medical conditions and will gain regulatory approval subsequently becoming integrated into evidence based treatment plans for various diseases, including mental health conditions.

Blockchain for Health Data Blockchain technology will play a role in securing and managing patient health data, ensuring privacy and data integrity. Patients will have more control over their data and consent for its use and sharing.

Healthcare Ecosystem Integration Digital health will be more seamlessly integrated into the broader healthcare ecosystem. It will allow the breakdown of organisational and departmental siloes. Electronic health records and interoperability will improve, allowing for the exchange of patient data between different providers and systems.

Virtual and Augmented Reality in Healthcare VR and AR will be used for medical training, patient education, and pain management. These technologies can also facilitate remote surgery and medical consultations.

Advanced Robotics Robotic technology is likely to play a more prominent role in future hospitals, assisting with surgery, patient care, and logistics. Surgical robots, pharmacy robots, robotic exoskeletons for rehabilitation, and robotic assistants for tasks like medication delivery could become more commonplace.

Mental Health Focus The importance of mental health and well-being will continue to gain recognition. Digital health solutions for mental health, including tele-therapy, meditation apps, and AI-driven mental health assessment tools, will proliferate.

Emphasis on Prevention and Wellness Healthcare systems will place a greater emphasis on preventive care and wellness programs to address health issues before they escalate. This shift could involve digitally enabled community outreach, education, and lifestyle interventions to promote healthier living.

Regulatory and Ethical Considerations As digital health innovations advance, regulatory bodies and ethical frameworks will need to evolve to address the unique challenges they present. Ensuring data privacy, security, and ethical use will remain crucial.

Global Expansion Digital health has the potential to bridge healthcare gaps in underserved regions, both domestically and globally. Telehealth and mobile health applications will expand access to healthcare services. It won't be long before we see an international virtual Hospital providing expert care from the developed to the developing world at scale.

The diagram below (Fig. 14.3), reworked from a paper by Butcher and Hussain [1] demonstrates the transition of digital health at a clinical level, with three

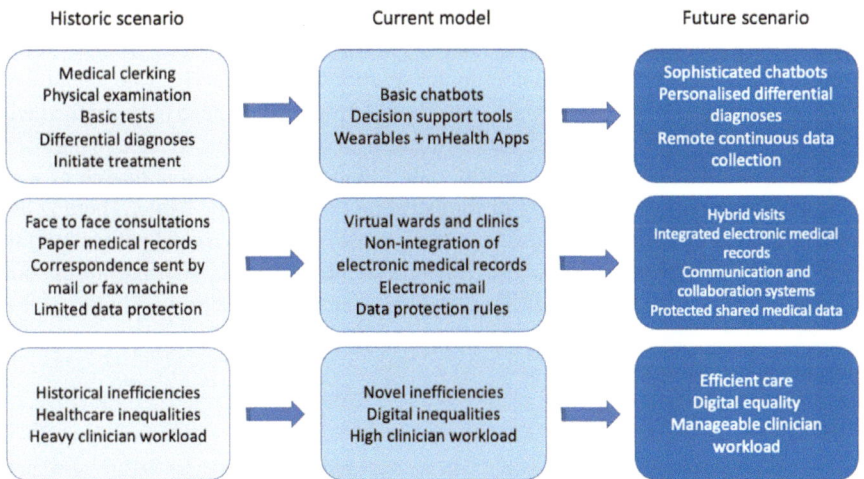

Fig. 14.3 Transitional model of digital health

segments presenting traditional care ('How it started'), current care ('How it's going') and a possible future care ('How it could be') paradigm.

Barriers and Moderators to Future Health

Patient Factors On the patient side there are several well-known issues which can impact on the potential uptake of digital health. These include demographic aspects such as; age, socio-economic status, education level and gender; technological poverty in terms of not having a smartphone or access to the internet at home, and individual level issues such as lack of motivation, lack of awareness and preference for in-person care. Many of these blockers are already being overcome. Over time, digital natives will become the elderly of tomorrow and already be familiar with using technology in all aspects of their lives. Even now we have the generation of silver-surfers who are keen to exploit the benefits of the internet but it is of course a priority to support more senior citizens to get online, to train them how to use web based systems and provide greater access through the loaning of digital devices and allowing access to remote monitoring systems, such as Birdie as we saw in Chap. 8, which have the major benefit of allowing people to remain independent in their own homes for longer. For those who simply do not wish to engage, then the mantra of 'digital first' but not 'digital only' will remain key.

The Healthcare Professional Most clinicians do already understand and appreciate the potential benefits of digital health to help them do their jobs. However, many are scarred by the experience of painful, slow and frustrating IT systems commonly used in healthcare settings, which frequently seem to hinder care delivery rather than enhance it. Technically challenged healthcare staff need to have regular and timely training, for example when a new EPR is rolled out, issues about poor technology design and interoperability need to be overcome by meaningful user engagement, along with assurances about the risks of information overload with smart new systems that require a degree in computer science to use properly. Some healthcare staff are very resistant to change, so new digital programmes need to be aligned with change management strategies and organisational development to make the most of the opportunities for service redesign, rather than the traditional approach of waiting for someone senior to retire or die before a change can be made. There is also the real concern about healthcare becoming more of a transactional process and the perception of impersonal care. This is a valid issue and needs to be part of the conversation about the process of change and service development well in advance of incorporating new technologies, otherwise we run the risk of losing the most meaningful aspect of care delivery.

Organisational Issues Within the system, be it in primary or secondary care, at a regional or national level, attention needs to be given to how digital solutions will be implemented. The many barriers include organisation size, flexibility, risk appetite and lack of dynamism at a management level. The costs and reimbursement, plus the age of existing legacy equipment and software need to be taken into account, plus a calculation about the real return on investment for a clever new clinical digital system. Many Hospital organisations will be concerned about licensing costs, the security of patient data (especially if they are outsourcing services into the cloud) and their legal liability if patient harm should arise as a consequence of a new technology. Over time, technology develops costs will go down but operating and maintenance costs will take a toll on business-as-usual budgets in already financially squeezed health systems. This means that cost-benefits analyses need to be robust and that implementation models (which are often poorly done) need to be well thought through and cost effective.

Conclusions

The future of digital health holds immense potential to improve patient outcomes, enhance healthcare delivery, and increase the efficiency of healthcare systems. However, it also raises important ethical and regulatory questions that need to be addressed to ensure responsible and equitable implementation. Additionally, as the field continues to evolve, stakeholders must remain vigilant in safeguarding patient privacy and data security. The recent pandemic has accelerated the move towards this future; however, important concerns remain. These include ensuring that new technologies are assessed effectively and are introduced thoughtfully, data is unified into care records, and, ultimately, digital tools are underpinned with appropriate clinical support. Patients must benefit without worsening workload for the clinician. Old barriers may be overcome but new challenges will be faced, in particular, ensuring the promise of better care for those who lack access to smart devices and the internet will be crucial.

To meet these concerns there is a strong case for a *Future Healthcare Institute*, as suggested by Harold Thimbleby in 2013 [4]. Which would be responsible for continually reviewing and prioritising new technologies and the principles of medical care to guide and align healthcare and new technological developments together. Such a body would understand the impact of digital health on patients and create legal, regulatory and ethical framework to support its safe implementation and ensuring that we are working together to solve the right problems in the right way, always incorporating our essential humanity.

It is not the strongest of the species that survives, nor the most intelligent, but the one most responsive to change.—Charles Darwin

References

1. Butcher CJ, Hussain W. Digital healthcare: the future. Future Healthc J. 2022;9(2):113–7. https://doi.org/10.7861/fhj.2022-0046.
2. Future Hospital Commission. Future hospital: caring for medical patients. 2013. http://www.rcplondon.ac.uk/sites/default/files/future-hospital-commission-report_0.pdf
3. Edwards N, Dunn S, Barach P, Vaughan L. The Wolfson Prize: designing the hospital of the future. Future Healthc J. 2023;10(1):27–30. https://doi.org/10.7861/fhj.2022-0105.
4. Thimbleby H. Technology and the future of healthcare. J Public Health Res. 2013;2(3):e28. https://doi.org/10.4081/jphr.2013.e28.

Further Reading

Tolf S, Mesterton J, Soderberg D, et al. How can technology support quality improvement? Lessons learned from the adoption of an analytics tool for advanced performance measurement in a hospital unit. BMC Health Serv Res. 2020;20:816.
Zimlichman E, Nicklin W, Aggarwal R, Bates DW. Health care 2020: the coming transformation. NEJM Catalyst. https://catalyst.nejm.org/doi/full/10.1056/CAT.20.0569

Index